Healing
Visualizations

BANTAM NEW AGE BOOKS

This important imprint includes books in a variety of fields and disciplines and deals with the search for meaning, growth, and change.

Ask your bookseller for the books you have missed.

Healing Visualizations

Creating Health
Through Imagery

Gerald Epstein, M.D.

BANTAM BOOKS
NEW YORK • TORONTO • LONDON • SYDNEY • AUCKLAND

This book is not intended as a substitute for medical advice of physicians. The reader should regularly consult a physician in matters relating to his or her health and particularly in respect to any symptoms that may require diagnosis or medical attention.

HEALING VISUALIZATIONS

A Bantam Book / August 1989

Bantam New Age and the accompanying figure design as well as the statement "the search for meaning, growth and change" are trademarks of Bantam Books, a division of Random House, Inc.

Library of Congress Cataloging-in-Publication Data

Epstein, Gerald, 1935–
   Healing visualizations.

      1. Imagery (Psychology)—Therapeutic use.
2. Self-care, Health. I. Title.
RC489.F35E635   1989   615.8'51   88-36251
ISBN 0-553-34623-7

Publishing simultaneously in the United States and Canada

PRINTED IN THE UNITED STATES OF AMERICA

CWO   15   14   13

For Rachel . . .
whose name means lamb

CONTENTS

ACKNOWLEDGMENTS

I wish to give special acknowledgments to some wonderful people who helped to make this book possible. First, I thank Harris Dientsfrey, an editor extraordinaire, whose diligent efforts and wise counsel helped bring this book to its final form. Of course the late Tobi Sanders, who initiated and molded Bantam's New Age division, is to be thanked for asking me to write this book.

Perle Besserman is to be thanked for her efforts in the beginning phase of this book, where she plowed through one thousand pages, editing the material to bring it to manageable shape.

Special thanks to Mme. Colette Aboulker-Muscat, my teacher in imagination, whose teachings pervade my understanding and conveying of imagery.

Ginny Flint is owed special thanks for her yeoman work in providing the drawings that dot the book. And, of course, how could there be a manuscript without the special typing efforts of Carol Shookhoff and Lisa Wood?

My thanks also to Leslie Meredith, who had the difficult task of taking over the book—after Ms. Sanders's untimely death—and seeing it through to completion. And to Rachel Blumenthal, who provided ceaseless support, encouragement, and suggestions all the way through.

I thank all the people who helped create a few of the imaging exercises, including Sheryl Rosenberg, Greta Gruber, Jean Kadmon, Dr. Andrew Gentile, and Dr. Viviane Lind, as well as my patients, who prefer anonymity.

To all of the above, I offer my most grateful thanks and appreciation.

INTRODUCTION

The Power of Imagery

In the early summer of 1974, I spent six weeks in Jerusalem as a visiting professor in law and psychiatry at Hadassah Medical School. At that time I was a practicing Freudian psychoanalyst. I was a traditionally trained medical doctor specializing in psychiatry and had gone on to become a psychoanalyst. Such a career had been my ideal since I was 19, and I realized it at 37. When I went to Jerusalem, I thought I had learned incontrovertible "facts" about the mind and had in my grasp the most central answers about mental life. In Jerusalem that summer, however, my understanding of the mind and of the profound connections between mind and body were transformed. One result is this book. It is the result of more than fifteen years of successful clinical practice using the vast imaginal powers of the mind to heal both physical and emotional disorders and to chart a course of health and heightened well-being.

In Jerusalem I met a young man who had undergone three years of extensive psychoanalysis—five times a week—to rid himself of persistent depression. His analysis had produced little relief. After these fruitless three years, he went

1

to a woman who practiced "visual imagery" or, more precisely, "waking dream" therapy. He had had four sessions with her—once a week, for a period of a month—and considered himself cured.

Given my Freudian perspective, I could hardly believe him. However, the fact remained that in one month, with a new and different kind of therapy, his depression had lifted.

My interest deeply aroused, I met with his therapist, Mme. Colette Aboulker-Muscat (a contemporary, I was later to find, of the French clinician Robert Desoille, who developed the imagery technique called "directed waking dream"). This meeting changed my life. I told Mme. Aboulker-Muscat that I had heard about her remarkable success with the young man but had never heard of her therapeutic technique. As we exchanged a few remarks about mental imagery, I recalled, and told Mme. Aboulker-Muscat, that Freud's explanation to analysts about using "free association" in essence was an imagery exercise. In Freud's exercise, the analyst tells the patient to *imagine* the two of them riding on a train, the patient looking out the window and describing to the analyst everything he or she sees.

Mme. Aboulker-Muscat responded by asking, "In what direction does the train go?" I was caught short by this seeming *non sequitur*. What did this have to do with therapy? Worried that somehow I would give the "wrong" answer, I cautiously said that trains go in a horizontal direction, and I made a horizontal gesture with my hand. Mme. Aboulker-Muscat made an upward movement with her hand and forearm, saying, "Well, what if the direction were changed to this axis?"

Now, some fifteen years later, I cannot detail what went through my mind at that moment. I am not sure that I knew then. What I did know, and still know as the truth of that moment, is that I felt an overwhelming sense of self-recognition, what is called an "aha" experience. It was an epiphany. The vertical movement seemed to lift me from the horizontal hold of the given, the ordinary patterns of everyday cause and effect. I leapt into freedom, and I saw that the task of therapy—the task of being human—was to help realize freedom, to go beyond the given, to the newness that we all are capable of, and to our capacity to renew and re-create. This is what imagery, I have come to learn, makes possible.

For the next nine years I studied with Mme. Aboulker-Muscat as an apprentice in imagination. I learned the unity of mind and body, mental and physical, and the therapeutic techniques of waking dream therapy, which enabled me to help my patients directly address and utilize the bodymind unity. Waking dream therapy is a deep experiential journey of inner life, using a person's night dreams or daily conversation as the starting point for waking exploration. The imagery exercises in this book are a form of waking dreams—dreams that can make reality.

What is mental imagery? Simply put, it is the mind thinking in pictures.

There are numerous ways we can think. Most familiar to us is logical thought. Since the seventeenth century, this type of thinking has been given precedence over all others because it is the basis of science. However, there are other forms of thinking—nonlogical, intuitive forms—which co-exist with logical thought. Consider when you have a flash of insight—when suddenly you see a new way to do something, have a new understanding, or find a solution to a problem that seemed to have no answer. This kind of thought is called intuition. As the educator Caleb Gattegno has rightly suggested, without intuition we would not be able to think of anything new.

Mental imagery, like intuition, is a type of nonlogical thinking. Logical, discursive thinking is used for making contact with people in the everyday world and with what can be called objective reality. Mental imagery is the thinking used for making contact with our inner subjective reality. My experience as a clinician asking his patients to peer into their inner lives has shown me that images form this structure of inner life.

The language of images is most commonly experienced as night dreams or daydreams. Anyone familiar with imagery learns almost immediately that we can work with this language as easily as we can work with spoken language. Indeed, the ability to understand and communicate in the language of images probably precedes the ability to communicate with words. Becoming aware of the language of images essentially requires only that we turn our attention to it.

As we shall see, the most remarkable feature of imagery work is that it can be accompanied by physiological changes. The beneficial physical effects of imagery would not be so surprising if we commonly thought of the mental and physical aspects as comprising two sides of a mirror that we term *body*. But for three hundred years, Western medicine has separated the mind from the body. You may be surprised to learn that no other medical system in the history of the world, including Western medicine prior to the seventeenth century, makes such a distinction.

Today, Western medicine has tentatively begun to explore the connections between the mind and body. Behavioral medicine and psychoneuroimmunology are two examples of this effort. Many studies in hypnosis have demonstrated more directly the impact of the mental on the physical. Researchers have found, for example, that hypnotized subjects can either give themselves poison ivy or prevent themselves from getting it, can induce burns, and can remove warts.

Though Western medicine (and Western science) is reluctant to accept that the mind can alter the body, it already firmly believes the reverse—that the physical can affect the mental—and it regularly utilizes this connection. Tranquilizers, antidepressants, and anesthetics are all examples of this. Since it is obvious that the body can affect the mind, does it not stand to reason that the use of mental power, such as will or imagery, can affect the body?

My clinical experience of the past fifteen years has borne witness not only to the effect of mind on body but to the power of mental imagery to help heal the body. I have seen this healing power across a wide range of physical disorders and maladies. The conditions that I have successfully helped patients treat using mental imagery include rheumatoid arthritis, enlarged prostate, ovarian cyst, inflammatory breast carcinoma, skin rash, hemorrhoids, and conjunctivitis. A friend of mine used mental imagery to cure himself of carcinoma of the liver. He had been told by doctors in 1982 that there was little hope for him, even with the chemotherapy treatments they started him on. He decided to use imagery techniques together with his chemotherapy for two years and, after 1984, discontinued chemotherapy but continued his imagery work. Today, he is still the only known survivor of this condition on record at the Memorial Cancer Sloan-Kettering Center in New York.

While many reports about imagery's efficacy have been anecdotal, meaning firsthand personal reports, they are as relevant and authentic as data collected by natural scientific methods. It is worth noting that there are now two major natural scientific journals devoted to imagery research: *The Journal of Mental Imagery* (from Marquette University) and *Imagination, Cognition and Personality* (from Yale University).

The familiar adage goes: "There is nothing new under the sun." This old saying holds true for the seemingly new field of visual imagery.

The medical use of imagery has existed in many cultures around the world for centuries (in Tibet, India, Africa; among Eskimos and American Indians), in some cases for millennia. In the Western world, as medical practice evolved from its ancient sources in Egypt and on into biblical times, imagery was an essential technique and sometimes *the* essential medical treatment for physical ailments, until approximately 1650, when natural science and modern medical thinking began to assume dominance.

More recently, while Freudian psychotherapy was sweeping through much of Europe, England, and then America, an undercurrent of imagery usage went virtually unnoticed. It was practiced mostly in France, Germany, and Italy, by independent clinicians, the most well-known of whom was Carl Jung. These men, trained as physicians and psychologists, used their imagery methods mainly for treating emotional illness. The techniques they developed went by various names: directed waking dream (Robert Desoille), active imagination (Carl Jung), guided affective imagery (Hanscarl Leuner), psychosynthesis (Roberto Assagioli). Their work paved the way for developing the use of imagery to treat physical illness.

It is a little-known fact that the most influential figure of twentieth-century psychology, Sigmund Freud, the man who invented talking therapy, once successfully used imagery to treat a 14-year-old boy suffering from a physical tic—and he did it in only one session. What is especially ironic about this episode is that while this case, treated by non-analytic means, was completed and successful, there is not one successfully completed case of psychoanalytic treatment reported by Freud in the twenty-five volumes of his published writings; it was the *only* successful, completed treatment mentioned in the twenty-five volumes of Freud's published writing and the only time Freud used imagery as a therapeutic technique.

Here is the case as it was reported by Freud in 1899, in *The Interpretation of Dreams:*

A fourteen-year-old boy came to me for psycho-analytic treatment, suffering from *tic convulsif,* hysterical vomiting, headaches, etc. I began the treatment by assuring him that if he shut his eyes he would see pictures or have ideas, which he was then to communicate to me. He replied in pictures. His last impression before coming to me was revived visually in his memory. He had been playing at draughts with his uncle and saw the board in front of him. He thought of various positions, favourable or unfavourable, and of moves that one must not make. He then saw a dagger lying on the board—an object that belonged to his father but which his imagination placed on the board. Then there was a sickle lying on the board and next a scythe. And there now appeared a picture of an old peasant mowing the grass in front of the patient's distant home with a scythe.

Freud then offered the young man an interpretation of the symbols. But the important point in this context is Freud's technique—a technique of mental imagery. After this one treatment, Freud states, the boy's tic and other symptoms disappeared. Freud's use of imagery apparently ceased as well.

This book offers, for the first time, an adaptation of mental imagery work for use with both physical and emotional problems that cut across a vast array of common (and sometimes not so common) ailments. These exercises provide you with a starting point for participating in your own healing. I am not suggesting that you stop seeing your doctor or stop taking prescribed medication. What I offer is an additional method whereby you can take an *active* part in your health and in getting well.

The exercises here, I want to emphasize, are not coping exercises. They are not new ways to deal with current experiences. Instead, imagery provides a technique to generate *new* experiences. Instead of simply reacting to experiences, you create them—as you do in your life when you intentionally set a new goal.

The organization of the book is straightforward. First, I discuss the easy mental preparation for doing imagery, some of the concepts behind it, and the simple physical techniques required. Next, in the heart of the book, I provide imagery exercises to use for more than seventy-five physical and emotional disturbances, listed alphabetically. Following that are powerful imagery exercises to help you enhance or maintain your health. Then I list eight pointers to help you in developing your own imagery, a natural process for most people. Finally, I conclude with some brief comments on what seem to me the large-scale implications of imagery.

Basically, this is a handbook on how to use imagery to help heal yourself and to help create your own good health.

I would like to explain the meaning of this book by an analogy that, to me, closely resembles the reality of life. I look at our individual lives as gardens that need to be tended. We are all essentially gardeners entrusted with our own reality-gardens. As gardeners, we have special functions, primarily weeding, seeding, and, of course, harvesting.

Gardens that are full of weeds cannot be harvested properly. Weeds will overrun the seeds and prevent them from taking root and blossoming. Illness, disease, and negative beliefs are weeds that we have allowed to grow in our personal gardens. Emotions such as anxiety, depression, fear, panic, worry, and despair are also weeds. Negative beliefs and emotions are intimately connected with illness and disease. It is no surprise to anyone who recognizes the basic unity of the bodymind that researchers have found a correlation between negative emotions and lowered immunity. Similarly, positive beliefs bring us positive emotions such as humor, joy, and happiness, and researchers have shown that positive emotions are tied in with healthy immune responses.

Mental imagery is a technique for clearing out the old, negative weed-beliefs and replacing them with new, positive seed-beliefs. By becoming a gardener of your own reality, self-healing becomes possible.

Health concerns us all. I have often wondered why we turn over the essential task of self-preservation to outside authorities. Part of the answer certainly is that we have not previously had the tools to enable us to help ourselves. Mental imagery is one of these tools, and we can use it to tend our gardens and assume authority for ourselves. Once you become an active gardener, you will gain more power over your health than you likely ever thought possible.

This is the genuine hope, power, authority, and freedom that we can gain from mental imagery as I describe it in the chapters that follow.

CHAPTER ONE

Picture Your Health:
Preparing for Imagery Work

A friend of mine was suffering from a bad cold. "I feel awful, Jerry," he said. "Do you have an imagery exercise that can help me?"

This is the exercise I prescribed, which anyone can use to help get over a common cold. The exercise is called **The River of Life**.

Close your eyes. Breathe out three times to relax yourself. See your eyes becoming clear and very bright. Then see them turning inward, becoming two rivers flowing down from the sinuses into the nasal cavity and throat, their currents taking away all the waste products, soreness, and stuffiness. The rivers are flowing through your chest and abdomen, into your legs, and coming out as black or gray strands that you see being buried deep in the earth. See your breath coming out as black air and see your waste products emerging from below. Sense the rivers pulsating rhythmically through the body and see light coming from above, filling up the sinuses, nose, and throat, all the tissues becoming pink and healthy. When you sense both

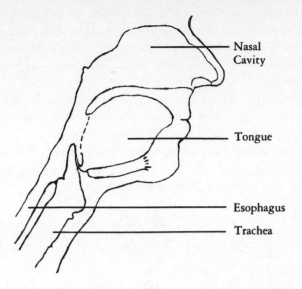

the rhythmic flow and the light filling these cavities, breathe out and open your eyes.

I told my friend to do this exercise every 3 hours for 3 to 5 minutes until his cold cleared up. Two days later, he reported to me that he had done the exercise for one day and promptly recovered.

A coincidence, many people would say. How could mental pictures about rivers and light have any effect on the physiological elements that trigger a cold? Don't colds get better by themselves anyway? Perhaps my friend's prompt recovery *was* a coincidence. However, for over fifteen years now I have regularly witnessed such coincidences in a wide variety of disorders, many of them far more serious than a cold.

I have chosen to begin with the example of my friend with a cold for two reasons—first, because a cold is one of the most common of physical ailments; second, because my friend's success shows that imagery work is extremely easy to do.

Friends have frequently asked me to suggest imagery exercises for use in all sorts of predicaments, crises, and illnesses, and they have regularly found the exercises useful. Imagery does not require subtle learning and extensive guidance.

Recently a friend of mine broke her wrist. It was set by an orthopedist, who told her that this particular bone required three months to heal. This diagnosis and prognosis was confirmed by a second orthopedist soon after the setting. I suggested that my friend help the healing along by using this exercise, **Weaving the Marrow.**

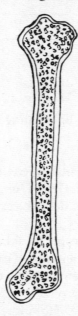

Close your eyes. Breathe out three times and see the ends of the bones as they now look. See the two ends touching each other. See and sense the marrow flowing from one end into the other. See this white marrow carried in blue channels of light flowing through the red bloodstream, seeing the arterioles flowing back and forth between the two ends, forming a woven net that brings the two ends closer. See the two ends knitting together perfectly until you can no longer see any sign of a break. Know that the bone is now one, and open your eyes.

I told her to repeat the exercise every 3 or 4 hours while she was awake, for up to 3 minutes each time. With this exercise, significant results should be seen in one to two weeks. After three weeks, my friend went to the orthopedist for a scheduled checkup, and the doctor found that the bone had healed. The orthopedist was so surprised that he immediately reexamined the X rays, which confirmed his original expectation: in his experience, the kind of bone that my friend had broken took three months to heal. The orthopedist could not explain the results he was seeing.

My friend told me that when she left the doctor's office, she was trembling with excitement at the realization of what she had done for herself.

Imaging—doing imagery—*is* a simple process. It means finding, discovering, or creating a mental picture, a mental *form*. This imagined—but still real—form has all the characteristics of any event, thing, or situation that we might see in everyday waking reality. The difference is that, unlike objects perceived when awake, they have no volume or mass. In short, they have no substance. Yet, they do have energy. We might think of these images as our mental children. We give birth to them to act on our behalf as agents of healing; then, with the energy they possess, they continue to stimulate the healing process on their own.

In discovering or creating these images, we are engaged in a meaningful process. The images are as real as our emotions and as meaningful as our night dreams. Obviously, what we create is a subjective reality, but it is a reality nonetheless, with the power to affect our bodies and to tell us more about who we are.

In this chapter we will discuss how to prepare our minds to do imagery and bring our inner reality to bear on our health. There is nothing very complicated in this. We use ordinary capacities available to all of us.

PREPARING THE MIND

There are four aspects to preparing our minds for imaginal healing. The first two are part of every imagery exercise. I call these elements *intention* and *quieting*. The second two are part of the imaging experience as a whole. I call these elements *cleansing* and *changing*.

Intention

Imaging is directly and dramatically connected to intention, the mental action that directs our attention and our actions. We all know about intention. "I intend to take my vacation next month," we say, and we plan accordingly. Intention guides us in matters large and small. When you turn on the television, it is because you intend to watch it. Intention is the active expression of our desires, channeled through our physiological systems. It often manifests itself as action— physical *or* mental action. Simply put, it is what we wish to achieve.

What does this have to do with imagery and healing? When we do an imagery exercise, we always begin by defining and clarifying our intention—what we want to achieve with the exercise. For example, if you want to heal a broken bone, you tell yourself before beginning the exercise that you are doing it to knit your bone. You are giving yourself an inner instruction. You might think of it as a kind of computer program for your mind, so that it focuses only on the process you're working on. When you tell yourself that you are going to accomplish a particular task, and when you are very clear about it, your success in using imagery will mount.

Intention depends on will, which is simply the life force impulse that enables us to make choices. We each have will, and it is reflected in the choices we make every day, all day, when we get up, put on our clothes, go to work, do our jobs—or read this book. All these actions are acts of will.

When we give our will a direction, then we have an intention. Intention is directed will, and it is essential to all self-healing work generated through the imagination. By using the imagination, we direct the will inward to find new pathways for ourselves, to take us to better health and richer lives. We become the conscious masters of our lives.

In the daily routine of life, we mostly use our wills to focus on external events: either we strive to get something from the world, or we strive to shape the outer world to our own needs (or to what we think are our needs). We forget that we can turn the same will, the same force of directed intention, toward ourselves to change and take charge of our lives. The alert will, the conscious intention, is at the center of imaginal healing. Often, we turn over the effort to help ourselves to others, to authorities of all kinds, because we have been conditioned *not* to use our wills for ourselves. Imaginal healing gives us the opportunity to achieve more independence and freedom. Some people might hesitate at taking this opportunity, but once they experience the benefits they are exhilarated rather than fearful. What such people need to remember is that they do no one, including themselves, any harm when they give themselves the freedom—the authority—to use their imaginations to contribute to their own healing.

Quieting

The second requirement for preparing our minds for imaginal healing is what I call quieting.

The healing environment requires two sorts of quieting: external and internal. External quiet helps us to concentrate on the task of moving inward. Distractions and everyday annoyances prevent this kind of attention. We do not require a monastery or a cave in order to image, but we do have to avoid the jarring effects of unsettling noises.

On the other hand, certain kinds of noises can help promote inner quiet: birds, the sounds of weather, even the distant hum of traffic (even honking!). If we do not become angry at the sounds or strain to ignore them, they will soon be part of the exercise. If you make active efforts to shut out the noise, you will be too busy attending to it, and you will "jam" the imagery process.

Some people have told me that they perform their exercises on the subway or on a public bus, which shows how teeming the setting can be! However, I do not recommend this practice (unless you are working on a disturbance for which you need to perform an exercise many times a day and are, perhaps, in a work setting) because it serves to incorporate imaginal work into the day's habitual activities. Imaging, as effortless as it is, is a special function, not another habit to add to your repertoire. Do not use imagery exercises as a diversion from the boredom of daily bus rides to work. The healing imagination has its own conditions, and it works best in a separate space and, for that matter, a separate time. In general, I recommend that imagery exercises be performed three times a day—before breakfast, at twilight, and before bed.

The inner aspect of quieting is relaxation. You may have noticed that the two imagery exercises I described earlier began with the instruction to breathe out. We shall talk more about the most useful way to breathe before beginning an imagery exercise, but here I want to point out that for the imaging work I prescribe, breathing out one or more times, as the case may be, is sufficient to create the appropriate degree of light relaxation.

Meditative or so-called deep relaxation is not appropriate here. In fact, it may make you less alert or even sleepy, and thus less responsive to the imagery experience. The focus is not to become relaxed but to image and remember. Attention, or heightened wakefulness, is the required state of mind, and imagery activity itself creates heightened attention.

Now, if you are generally quite tense and the breathing-out exercise is not sufficient to produce an inner relaxation, there is an additional relaxation exercise for you in chapter 5. But remember, "deep" relaxation is not desired.

Cleansing

A third aspect of imagery work is what I call cleansing. Not every imagery exercise involves cleansing, but cleansing is one of the most important first steps in opening yourself to becoming whole.

Most ancient medical systems employed cleansing procedures. Egyptian physicians, for example, made bathing a requirement for healing, as did all known cultures of the ancient world, East and West. The Romans were famous for their advanced bathing and purification techniques at their healing springs. The modern spa and European hydrotherapy are popular offshoots of that ancient cleansing process for inducing health. The ancient Jews instituted a purification ritual called *mikvah,* which was as much a reminder of the need for personal health as it was a celebration of the Sabbath (itself being a day of cleansing).

The general response to cleansing is felt as a sense of unburdening, which most of us experience at least to a small degree when we bathe or shower. Clinical experience confirms the inner meaning of cleansing. Consider the many moods and ailments associated with "darkness" and "dirt." Many acute epidemics of bacterial infections that decimated populations around the world originated in environments of deteriorated public health and unsanitary conditions. In our own times, chronic disease occurs in climates of increasingly polluted air, earth, and water.

Mental illness, including the psychotic states, are characterized by "dirty" thoughts such as violent sexual fantasies and guilt-associated acts like masturbation. People who are extremely depressed are often physically unkempt and, like psychotics, become increasingly dirty as they lose interest in social relations and lack the physical energy required to clean their bodies. An extreme, though increasingly common, example today are the unfortunate homeless people laden with bags of garbage, unrecognizable as either male or female under their coat of grime. The original meaning of insane was "unclean."

In saying that cleansing is necessary for imagery work, I am of course talking about more than physical cleanliness. Without being moralistic about it, I would suggest that to be healthy is to be "clean" in every sense of the word. Ethically speaking, we must ask ourselves how "clean" we are in our interactions with others. Many people expect to be free of disease as part of their birthright. Yet, they deceive themselves if they see no connection between illness and unscrupulous behavior, and the resulting experiences of guilt and self-punishment—even if they outwardly get away with their "dirty deeds."

How many times have we heard the expression, "The body doesn't lie"? In my experience, that applies as much to our moral and ethical health as to our eating habits, exercise, and attitudes toward work. For each of us, every moral or ethical indiscretion is registered in our bodies and can adversely influence the workings of our physical and mental lives.

An ethical indiscretion does not mean only that you are willfully cheating or harming someone else. The issue is more complex. You can cheat yourself, too.

A patient came to me suffering from cancer. Cancer had run through his family on his mother's side for about four generations. In each generation, moreover, a male sibling of the cancer victim behaved in such a way as to bring shame, disgrace, and disruption to the family. All of the cancer victims were the heads of their families and knew of the siblings' activities. They also chose to keep the matters to themselves, bearing their dismay and grief privately.

In the instance of my patient, the black-sheep sibling was a compulsive gambler who was heavily in debt and was running his family into the ground. My patient was taking money from his own family to try to pay off his brother's debts. His family was suffering and did not know why. My patient was, in effect, unwittingly stealing from his own family. Further, he was lying by not telling the entire family what was going on. His moral life was being compromised (he was an honest, upstanding man) because of his "support" of his brother's negative behavior.

In our work together, my patient came to see that he should inform the whole family of his brother's situation. When this was done, the air was cleared, and the rest of the family came to the sibling's aid by confronting him. As a result, he went into treatment, including Gambler's Anonymous.

As for my patient, he felt a burden lifted from him, and he began to enter a phase of remission.

To heal ourselves, we must begin by "cleaning up our act." This is part of the conscious act of will that precedes the opening of the imaginal eye, part of the decision to take a hard, clear inward look at ourselves and be open to understanding what our bodies and feelings are telling us. By using images, we can clear away our denials that something is wrong, clean up our delusions, and shine a light on our habitual destructive patterns. Then we can meet our ailments in person and heal ourselves. Cleansing is part of healing, and together they make space for new, healthful patterns to emerge, for new, positive growth and wholeness.

An imaginal cleansing exercise is also a wonderful way to prepare yourself for the day. You can find a cleansing exercise in chapter 5.

Changing

What do I mean when I say that changing is an element of healing through imagery?

Modern quantum physicists and Chinese mystics both have said that what we subjectively experience as time, our limited picture of reality, is actually the continuous flow of change. The entire traditional Chinese medical system is, in fact, based on the premise that illness is synonymous with blockages of flow—in other words, with resistance to the changing nature of things.

We try to hold on to what we think of as "good situations," and in our holding, we tighten up, resist the possibility of pain or nonpleasure, and so run head-on into the very pain we are trying to avoid. It is logical that the act of holding on to something impermanent, pretending that it is permanent, must lead to trouble. Most often, the form the trouble takes is a physical ailment.

Everyone I know who has worked with imagery reports that "feeling better" comes with "letting go"—of things, ideas, preconceptions about themselves or others—with dropping their effort to stop the flow of life's events. They don't become fatalists and passively sit by the river, saying "what will be, will be." Rather, they actively let go of the desperation involved in identifying themselves with fixed, limited experiences, things, and situations. As the process of letting go deepens, so does the sense of well-being. Imagery and flowing with the process of change are inextricably linked.

This may be due to a function of the left-right–brain phenomenon—the fact that the right brain seems connected with intuition and picture-making, while the left brain seems connected with functions of logic, words, and rational thought. Giving free rein to the imagination, to acausal pictures rather than to sequential word-thinking, enables us to yield to the flow of things. When we restore the imagination to its place of equality with logical thinking, we open ourselves to change and renewal. We give ourselves a chance to enjoy the constant succession of now-moments as they unfold.

This is quite the opposite of our usual experience, in which we most often concentrate on the past or the future. When we do this, we are focusing on discontinuity rather than on flow. We connect ourselves to fixed points to which we attach a damaging kind of judgment and significance.

For example, we think of ourselves as "graduating from high school on June 7, 1953," or we say that "the attack on Pearl Harbor took place on December 7, 1941," and then we attach to these events a set of thoughts, memories, feelings, projections, and attitudes. The events become hardened little souvenirs, and we surround ourselves with them, in a shell-like fashion, a shell that over time becomes harder and harder to break through in the normal course of life. If we could just note the event itself, without any commentary, without the kind of personalizing or judging or liking or disliking that human beings are so accustomed to, we would not get stuck with the "feeling identifications" that can bring about illness and the distemper of unhappiness. Not that we might stay youthful and healthy forever, but that we might age with the graceful flexibility we so admire in saints and heroes, who are really no different from the rest of us—except for their heightened ability to flow with life's changes.

Once we are attuned to change, we can recognize the paradox that many of us live. Most of us tend to regard ourselves as individualistic, seemingly independent, resourceful beings who act to shape our own destinies. Yet, at the same time, we usually are deeply afraid of appearing "different" from others. Although it is deeply satisfying to think of ourselves as independent, in reality we are often resistant to new ways of looking at things, which is the real hallmark of individuality and independence. We like to see ourselves as different from and more self-determined than other people, and indeed this may be so. But for some of us, this feeling may hide a craving for social approval—that is, sameness.

In the material world we strive to stand out by becoming richer, more "self-made" than others, but as we rise in the world, we find ourselves conforming to the norms of other rich people. Granted, there is more freedom to indulge your fancy when you have money, but wealthy people can become just as bored with their lives of luxury as the rest of us can become tired from the effort to earn money. Change does not take place in people who alter merely their outward circumstances.

Imaginal work on our bodies and minds is a start in the process of freeing ourselves to become true individuals, so that we may live easily with change. By enabling us to turn away from the fixed world of goods and appearances, imaginal work helps us discard the constrictive behavior and attitudes that often adversely affect our health.

Intention, quieting, cleansing, changing—these are the components of a healing state of mind. You will find each of these activities rewarding in and of itself. As you read further, and learn how to use these components to help heal your particular ailments and problems, you will become not only a healthier person but a freer one, ready to experience some of the infinite possibilities that life offers us.

CHAPTER TWO

The Imaging Process:
The Mind-Body Connection

What goes on in our minds and our bodies when we do imagery work? How does an "insubstantial" phenomenon such as imagery alter the substance of our bodies? As I have already noted, research science has not examined the phenomenon of healing through imagery in a thorough and methodical manner, although certain studies have demonstrated a definite mind-body link. But we can draw on clinical experience, the workings of our lives, and the insights of other cultures to gain an understanding of the imagery process.

EMOTIONS, SENSATIONS, AND IMAGES

The key to the process of imagery work lies in the connections between emotions, sensations, and images.

Let us start with emotions. People commonly think of emotions as consisting only of feelings such as happiness, anger, satisfaction, and sadness. I see emotion more broadly, as our movement to stimuli. Emotion literally means "movement from." Therefore, emotion equals movement, and movement is the essence of life, our élan. Sometimes our movements take the form of inner feelings such as happiness, anger, satisfaction, and sadness, feeling states that have duration over time and that reverberate within us; sometimes they take the form of physical action or reactive outbursts such as displays of anger or surprise, which are discharged immediately. To my way of thinking, there is no life without emotion—that is, without the movement experienced in response to stimuli. Emotion is life, and emotion has both the outward form of action or reaction and the inward form of feeling.

Emotions are intimately connected with images. Every emotion can manifest itself as an image. There is a simple way you can prove this to yourself. Simply ask yourself to "see" any feeling that you have. If you are happy, ask yourself what your happiness looks like; if you enjoy sports, ask yourself what your enjoyment looks like; if you do not like stupidity, ask yourself what stupidity looks like. In every case, I assure you, an image will come to you. This is *your* image. No one else in the world has precisely the same image. It is the visual form of your feeling. Images give form to emotions.

In my fifteen years of clinical experience working with imagery, I have not found a single person capable of imaging who was unable to call forth an image of his or her feeling.

An image is the mental form of a feeling. But there is also a physical form—sensations. A feeling has certain physical sensations associated with it. When you are angry, for example, you often experience a constriction in your chest. When you are happy, you often experience a sense of lightness throughout your body. Just as a feeling has physical sensations associated with it, so does an image. There are no images without accompanying sensations.

In imagery work, you use your images to change your emotions or your sensations. In essence, you use images to create and affect your experience. This is how you do it: As you work on your images and change them, you simultaneously change and create the sensations and emotions that accompany them. Once the image changes, so does the emotion, and so do the sensations. Like the sides of an equation, emotion and image are equal, two expressions of the same reality, and sensation is attached to both. When you change the image, you change the whole equation. Then you will see that images are indeed a road to good health, both physical and mental.

THE VERTICAL AXIS OF IMAGERY

My experience with Mme. Aboulker-Muscat revealed to me that imagery work takes place outside the mechanistic realm of cause and effect. It takes place, in a manner of speaking, above the earth. When Mme. Aboulker-Muscat asked me to identify the direction of a train, I made a horizontal gesture. When she then turned her arm upward, creating a vertical axis, and asked me what would happen if a train moved along that axis, I saw that the train would be free of ordinary cause and effect. It would be above the earth.

I believe that imagery work takes place in the vertical axis.

In the ordinary world of cause and effect, everything is fixed and repetitive. There is no newness. Such-and-such an action always causes such-and-such a reaction. So many particular proteins strung together in a particular chain always form the same particular amino acid. Such-and-such quantities of certain chemicals always produce the same substance. The world of Newtonian physics is the ordinary world of cause and effect.

But the human realm is different from the realm of

physics. We live in a world that we make, physically, emotionally, psychologically—a world in the vertical axis. And when we do imagery, we recognize that human life obeys more than ordinary cause and effect. We have the capacity to make something new—and to influence the physical material of our own bodies. If we were just mechanisms, then of course only a mechanic could hope to change us. But we are more than this and can change ourselves.

Imagery work always attempts to put people on the vertical axis, which escapes gravity as it moves upward and enables a person to escape the ordinary constrictions of earth-bound living. In the exercises in this book, you regularly will find yourself on the vertical axis. When you begin to develop your *own* images for self-healing, I believe that you again will frequently find yourself moving upward, then downward as you complete the exercise. One example: A friend called and explained in passing that he had viral conjunctivitis. I suggested that he imaginally take his eyes out of their sockets, wash them in healing waters, and put blue light in the sockets. Several days later, when we spoke again, he reported that his eye had begun improving once he started the exercise. But why, he asked me, did he always find himself moving upward to get to the healing waters? I explained that moving upward was the direction of freedom, and healing. My friend, by himself, had discovered the vertical axis. (He also reported that after he returned his eyes to the blue-light-filled sockets, the dark-green lush vegetation around the healing waters had burst into flowers!)

Given my experience with imagery, it did not surprise me to learn, as I studied other medical systems, that all cultures and traditions have linked upward movement with transcendence, with myths of flight, with severing the bonds and limitations of everyday habitual behavior and activity and finding new paths, new ways of being.

REMEMBERING YOURSELF

When we think about healing, we are thinking about becoming whole. Becoming whole means putting ourselves back together, and when we are ill, we have, to some extent, fallen apart. Healing means that we have come back to our unity.

The model for the healing function of becoming whole was portrayed more than five thousand years ago in ancient Egypt in the story about the god Osiris, who was murdered by his brother Seth. His body was dismembered into fourteen pieces, each piece buried in a different part of Egypt. Osiris's wife Isis *re-collected* these hidden pieces and brought Osiris back to life by *re-membering* him, by putting all the pieces together.

Remembering literally means to reconnect one piece of the body to another. The body means physical and mental and emotional. Putting ourselves together includes all three. Remember also means to recall. Remembering, then, is to restore ourselves to wholeness by recalling our unity and putting our bodymind back together. Imagery is the mental way of remembering and recalling. The act of seeing in pictures is to see in wholes and is the mental analogy to physical remembering.

If health and wholeness are associated with remembering, then it follows that illness is associated with forgetting. When we have lost our unity, which is what illness tells us has happened, then we have forgotten ourselves. Surgery may be an attempt to re-member on a physical level. Imagery is the analogous process on the mental level—and can effect remembering on the physical level.

In ancient times, philosophers such as Plato saw the individual as a little world that was a smaller version of the national and cosmic worlds. The imaginal doctor is in line with this holistic tradition. Any rupture in the link between the individual and the greater world—the world of the family or the even greater world of the social realm—requires repair along the entire line. When an individual re-members his or her personal history, a positive "ripple effect" occurs, contributing ultimately to restructuring the entire family of humankind.

This is where imaginal therapy ends and healing, in the sense of unifying, begins; where "patient" becomes "person," reaching beyond cure of symptoms toward total self-renewal; where a doctor can and need no longer be a guide.

CARING AND CURING

Cure means the end of symptoms. The first step in the curing process is taken when you begin *caring* for yourself. Imaginal medicine strongly emphasizes that you help heal yourself, that you become your own healer to the extent that this is possible. (Obviously, if, say, you break your leg, you should not necessarily believe that all you need are a few doses of imagery to repair the leg.) The practice of mental imagery is meant to help you discover and use your own inherent resources, to give you the tools that allow you to help cure yourself and to augment what you are doing if you are under the guidance of your doctor.

I have found that I help my patients best by striking a creative spark in them and allowing them to find their own ways of maintaining balance in themselves. I do not cure my patients; only they can cure themselves. I teach patients imagery exercises, thereby giving them the tools to help to care for themselves. It is then up to the patients to create their own medicine in the act of administering it.

When someone is being guided in imaginal work, the situation is not unlike a conversation carried on in the language of pictures. Patient and guide are engaged in an active collaboration in which each act of the patient's imaging necessitates that the guide be equally active in "receiving" the images. The effect of the imager's full involvement is that the imager remembers both the inherent information in and the power of the images that he or she has voluntarily called forth as a tool for healing. And all this is accomplished in ordinary waking states of mind, without any further help from the guide. The imager is encouraged to remember the image and what it suggests, not to forget it and wait for some outside situation or subliminal cue to stimulate it into action.

In imaginal medicine, when my instruction ends, you turn from patient into self-healer. Like physical exercise, imaginal workouts are more effective when practiced regularly. Their benefits are both immediately rewarding and cumulative, bringing a new balance into the disorder from which you have been suffering.

Keeping up this new order is your responsibility, and it is an ongoing job. People who have a creative imagination and the discipline to use it in a structured fashion on a regular basis are better able to maintain the order and balance in their lives than are people who would rather lie back (literally) and let a doctor or therapist do their healing for them. But *anyone* can learn to use imaging techniques effectively. Once you let your imagination work for you, you will find yourself feeling more hopeful and positive because of the inner light of imagination shining into your existence.

This hope is realistic. The difference between wishful thinking and realistic hope is that wishful thinking usually has some negative experience associated with it, such as doubt or anxiety. Realistic hope has no such negative current. It is a sober appraisal and often provides a sense of peace.

Some patients do not want to enter into more equal relationships with their doctors. They cling to their old dependencies, finding it more convenient to rely on outside help for their succor. The alienated and lonely find that their contact with doctors is one of their only human relationships. They sustain this contact by staying in the role of sick patient dependent on a doctor for survival. They feel so helpless and so depleted of energy that they want the doctor to do all the work, without taking any responsibility for their own healing. But imagery can help even these patients discover inner reservoirs of strength.

Over and over again I have tried to show people how important it is for them to help themselves. Of course I understand that when someone is in pain, a "quick fix" is hard to pass by. Aspirin works quickly to make a headache disappear and let you go about your business. But when you explore the pain with the inner eye of your imagination, you discover the meanings expressed in the pain, and you can cure it on both the mental and physical levels of your bodymind. These results are, of course, more long-term and more profound then those provided solely by taking pills.

THE MIND-BODY SPLIT

Throughout this book there will be frequent references to the "bodymind." As you may know, a large number of people, including most doctors and scientists, do not regard body and mind as one unit. From the mid-seventeenth century on, science has treated the physical body as an autonomous entity having little or nothing to do with the mind or the emotions. Even Freud, who helped underscore the power of the emotions, and modern-day psychologists share this prejudice. To oversimplify: medical doctors say that only the body exists; psychologists say that emotions exist but they see no integral connection between the emotions and the physical substance of the body.

In the process of intellectually splitting the body from the mind, each has been broken down into tinier and tinier units, so that rigid medical specialties have sprung up to deal with disorders of the ear, foot, brain, psyche, and so on. In reality, there has never been a mind-body split, nor can there ever be. Body and mind are two aspects of the same human experience: the body is quantitative, the mind is qualitative. Thus, even if a clinician cannot locate a physical disturbance to explain your physical complaint, and says to you, "It's all in your mind," there is still a physical event going on. If it is in your mind, it is in your body too. They are analogies of each other.

THE EMOTIONAL-PHYSICAL MIRROR

The perspective of bodymind enables us to see that physical symptoms are a reflection, a mirroring, of emotional issues; the physical symptoms are directly connected to the emotions. That is, the body is both physical and emotional. These two components are as two sides of a coin, inseparable, although one may be hidden from our sight while the other visibly manifests itself.

To view the physical and the emotional as operating together can be enormously beneficial to you, because the more that is disclosed to you about yourself, physical or emotional, the more control you have over yourself.

Take the case of the man who came to see me suffering from coronary insufficiency, so that he easily became short of breath and fatigued. He had previously undergone open-heart surgery and had taken it upon himself to exercise and to eat differently. Still, he felt troubled. He complained of feeling sad and depressed, in addition to his physical symptoms. In discussing with me how he felt about his life, he discovered that he was *heartbroken* because he thought his wife did not love him. Here was the key. The man's melancholy had not caused the heart condition, nor had his heart condition caused the melancholy. Both his emotional state and his physical condition were expressions of his distress over his marriage and lack of love from it. This was the context in which his disturbance was making itself known. This disturbance was an *effect* of a broader disturbance in the man's life. The open-heart surgery had dealt with one effect of the disturbance. Now he had to confront the contextual cause of his illness.

Every part of the physical body has its emotional counterpart. When we perceive this emotional meaning, we give ourselves a larger context in which to relate to our bodies. This means that each symptom or syndrome has a source to which the symptom is drawing our attention. Without this knowledge, we usually pay minimal attention to the process of healing, other than to rid ourselves of the bothersome symptom.

Often, if the symptom is not too troublesome, we do nothing about it, and it clears up over time. On these occasions, the educational opportunity provided by illness has been wasted. Fortunately or unfortunately, depending on one's viewpoint, the symptoms often reappear even more intensely, and our bodymind offers us yet another opportunity to understand more clearly who we are.

In the listings of disturbances in chapter 4, I shall try to indicate something about the context and meaning of each symptom as I outline imagery exercises for the common troubles we face. Much of our physical-emotional imbalances concern significant relationships, or moral and ethical questions. Looking at these factors frequently helps to bring about relief. You are likely to find that in doing some of the imagery exercises I outline, a number of these social or interpersonal issues spontaneously spring to your attention. Let your body and mind speak to you, and allow yourself to listen.

CHAPTER THREE

Practicing Successful Imaging:
The Path to Wholeness

Imaging succeeds in direct proportion to how successfully you can turn your senses away from the outside world and toward the inner realm. Turned inward, you can create a mental image that can stimulate your physical body. The image will come to you on its own as long as you direct your will and attention inward, away from the outer world.

BODY POSTURE FOR IMAGING

The most effective body position for imaging is to sit in what I call the Pharaoh's Posture: sitting upright in a straight-backed chair that has armrests, with your back straight, your arms resting comfortably on the armrests, and your hands open, palms down or up as it suits you. Your feet should be flat on the floor. Neither your hands

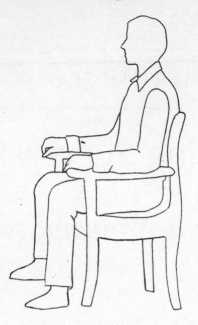

nor your feet should be crossed during the period of imaging, nor should they come into contact with any other part of your body. This arrangement of hands and feet is part of the technique of keeping our sensory awareness focused away from external stimuli.

Throughout the ages, the Pharaoh's Posture was assumed by royalty who sought their inner guides before making a decision. It is a posture expressing the search for inner guidance.

A straight-backed chair is best because a straight spine permits a sense of awareness to infuse our attention. Lying down, in either a horizontal or a reclining position, is associated with sleeping, and it reduces the heightened awareness required for imaging sharply.

Sitting with your back straight also enhances your breathing; your lungs need this vertical posture in order to expand fully. And awareness of breath, as all ancient physicians and healers knew, promotes greater alertness and attentiveness to mental processes. We become more attuned to our inner life as we become more conscious of our breathing.

While the Pharaoh's Posture is ideally suited to imaging, there are instances in which imagery has to be done instantly—for example, when one is experiencing anxiety. In these situations, imaging may be done standing up, wherever you may be.

BREATHING FOR IMAGING

Breathing plays an essential role in all inwardly directed experience. Those who meditate become relaxed and quiet by counting their breaths. The Chinese equate breath with the mind itself. Yoga exercises, natural childbirth, weight lifting, running, or any other sport involving concentrated intention, all focus on breath.

Most of us are not generally aware of our breathing. We are not usually comfortable directing ourselves to our inner life. We are an active people with the urge to conquer the outside world and take mastery over nature. But the inner life holds the cure to our physical and emotional imbalances and the promise of harmony between body, mind, and spirit. Breathing is the starting point that allows the inward turning to occur; it is the link that enables us to discover our personal imagery.

To enhance the presence of images, tell yourself to become quiet and relaxed (your intention). Breathe rhythmically, in through the nose and out through the mouth. The exhalations through the mouth should be longer and slower than the inhalations, which are normal, easy, without effort—that is, not labored or exaggerated. Breathing out longer than breathing in stimulates the major quieting nerve in the body, the vagus. Originating at the base of the brain, in the medulla, this nerve extends down through the neck and sends branches to the lungs, heart, and intestinal tract.

Under the influence of enhanced exhalation, the vagus plays a role in lowering blood pressure, slowing the pulse, heart rate, and muscular contractions of the intestinal tract, and reducing the respiratory rate. When these functions are quiet, your attention is more fully available for imagery work.

I stress exhalation over inhalation because breathing to quiet the body begins with an *out*breath, not an *in*breath. The usual way of in-out breathing stimulates us by exciting our sympathetic or excitatory nervous system and the adrenal medulla, which secretes adrenaline. Out-in breathing, on the other hand, stimulates the parasympathetic nervous system and the vagus nerve, which help the body quiet down and relax.

When you are comfortable with your breathing and feel ready to begin your imagery work, instruct yourself to *breathe out three times* (or two times, or one time as the case may be). This may sound odd but is quite simple. You breathe out, then in; out, then in; then out again—for a total of three outbreaths and two inbreaths. After this you begin your imagery exercise, breathing regularly.

During your work, your attention will be focused on the images, and your breathing will take care of itself. When the imaginal event is ended, you may take one outbreath before opening your eyes.

It will take you only a few seconds to establish this reverse breathing pattern. Exhaling first and inhaling second will become second nature once you have learned to image.

IF AT FIRST YOU CAN'T IMAGE

Obviously, not everyone has the same capacity for imaging. For most, the process comes easily, almost at once. Others may need to devote more practice time before imaging comes readily to them.

Here are a few tips to stimulate your capacity for imaging.

If you experience difficulty in doing the exercises in this book, look at pictures or photographs of natural settings for 1 to 3 minutes, then close your eyes and try to see the same pictures in your mind. Another approach is to remember a pleasant scene from your past, with your eyes open. Then close your eyes and try to re-create each detail of the scene. You can also use your nonvisual senses. For example, hear fish frying in a skillet or the applause of an audience or glasses clinking; try using perfumes or essences of varying strengths to evoke images.

If you continue to have trouble, you may not be using— may not be noticing—the images that come to you. You might be sensing something auditory or somatic (bodily senses) or kinesthetic (body position), yet not *see* these images. What sense do you use or respond to most easily? For example, if you're an auditory person, hear the sound of the ocean and see what images come up from that. When you consciously focus your attention on what you are sensing, you can slip gently from that mode into the connected visual image. All the senses are connected and become visual once you ask yourself to describe your experience.

Some people have the habit of verbalizing rather than visualizing, turning images quickly into words. If this applies to you, practice looking around at your environment for a few minutes without naming, labeling, or categorizing what you see. Or look at an image in a book or magazine, then cover it and try to recall what you just saw by describing it rather than by naming it. If you reflexively start to name things, just return, without blaming yourself, to seeing.

In general, when trying to improve your imagery, make an effort to relax (breathe out deeply three times and close your eyes), and let the imagery come—that is, *wait for it.* And when it comes, accept it. Whatever appears is right and can be useful, even if it seems silly or impossible.

While you may take some time to activate imagery at the beginning, you will need less time with practice.

OBTAINING RESULTS

Make an effort to try your imagery exercises regularly or as
recommended in each exercise. But do not make a concerted
effort to get results. This "undemanding" approach might
be difficult for you at first. Many of us are concerned
primarily with results—we see them as the most important
aspect of life. This is not the case when it comes to healing.
Keep your focus squarely on the *process* of imagery and on
your *intention* to heal. The more you worry about getting
well, the more difficult you will make the healing process
for yourself.

The action of healing takes place in the present instant.
Directing your attention to the past or the future (to outcome and results) takes you away from the field of action.
As soon as you concern yourself with the outcome, you will
naturally begin to feel anxious or scared or worried, or all
three. Thinking about the past often brings feelings of
guilt, depression, and regret. Any of these feelings will
immediately take you away from the task at hand, and your
concentration on your healing will be broken.

In our imaging as in our lives, we must do our share, and
we also must allow the universe to do its part. We certainly
control our beliefs about what we do *in* and *to* the universe,
but that is all the control we have. After that, we can only
listen, wait, and be patient for a response.

Even if you are suffering and desperately want to feel
better, do not anticipate results. Have you not noticed that
the more you desire results, the more your suffering in-
creases? When your hopes do not materialize, you feel
disappointed and even more hopeless, and your condition
worsens. Take heart, though: if you leave the results to
"heaven," you will experience relief, if not complete healing, in a relatively short time. But do not ask how long it
will take. Forget the outcome for the moment. Just take
responsibility for your own effort and do your part.

If you cannot leave the results to heaven, here is a simple way to help yourself. Notice when you have expectations and see yourself cutting the expectation with a pair of scissors or tossing it over your shoulder into the sea, or see the expectation going like a balloon into the sky.

Imagery is one of the best methods for strengthening our faith and trust in ourselves. Take the case of "Jennifer," a young woman who came to see me for a problem of infertility. Previous tests had shown her to have normal fallopian tubes. Under my instruction, she did imagery work with the intention of becoming pregnant (an exercise for infertility is in chapter 4) and discovering the physical trouble that was preventing conception. Jennifer's imagery exercise revealed that the end of one fallopian tube near the ovary was sealed, crusted over by adhesions and scar tissue, the origin of which she could not explain. Nevertheless, if her imaging was accurate, she had uncovered a physical-mechanical incapacity of her fallopian tubes. She said nothing to her gynecologist about this, since she felt he would not believe her. She tried cleaning her fallopian tubes imaginally.

Eventually, she decided to have a fallopian tube transplant, in which an egg is fertilized in the fallopian tube through a surgical procedure. When her lower abdominal region was opened for this surgery, Jennifer's fallopian tube was found to be in *exactly* the condition she had discovered through imagery, although no physical tests (including a sonagram) had revealed this.

After the operation, Jennifer was awed and amazed to find that she knew more about herself than did her doctors. She immediately felt increased confidence in her intuition and grew more trusting of her judgment.

Of course we know more about ourselves than anyone else can! All we need is the trust it takes to believe this. In Jennifer's case, one successful imaginal experience was enough to encourage her belief and trust in herself.

LENGTH OF EXERCISES

The rule of thumb for imaginal medicine is that *less is more*. The shorter the imagery, the more powerful it is.

It does not take long to experience a sensation. When you have felt a sensation, the imagery has done its work. If you don't feel some sensation or emotion after a relatively short period of time, do not strive after it by extending your work with that particular image. Instead, try another image.

What sensations might you feel? They vary from person to person and problem to problem. The sensations include twitching, pulsation, heat, itching, pain, tingling, a buzz, and so on.

Many of us tend to think that more effort brings more results, but imagery works in the opposite way. In performing imaginal healing, we use a small jolt—a seed, as it were—to stimulate our own powerful responses.

Most exercises in this book take from 1 to 5 minutes. Many people feel that this is less than they could or should be doing, particularly when their ailments are serious. Their anxiety often creates the idea that they must "spare no effort." But the constant application of effort simply is not necessary in imagery work. Once an initial imagery exercise has been accomplished, we need only little reminders to stimulate the body's recollection of healing activity. Imagery needs to be practiced, but it should not become an obsession. One trigger is all we need to promote the physiological mechanisms that aid bodily repair. Pavlov conditioned dogs to salivate at the sound of a bell. Through imagery, we condition ourselves to stimulate healing processes with a mental picture. In this analogy, the image corresponds to the bell as the stimulus, and the healing process corresponds to the salivation.

The following story provides an example of a trigger that sets loose a powerful physiological effect. I learned of it while working in an alcohol clinic in a New York hospital.

A group of thirty former heroin and methadone addicts, who had been free of drugs for ten years, agreed to participate in an experiment in which they would board a bus that would take them to 125th Street in New York City, where, a decade earlier, they had bought their drugs. The moment the bus reached the corner where they had once made their purchases, the ex-addicts went into a state of drug withdrawal. The image was only a street corner, but it was sufficient to stimulate a disproportionately strong negative physical response.

For an example of a strong positive reaction to a minute stimulus, simply think of a grandparent who hears the name of his or her grandchild.

Age can be a factor in determining the amount of the imaginal "dosage." As we get older and our habits become more deeply ingrained, it becomes more difficult to create new habits and to experience our reactions to them—which is precisely what repairing ourselves is. As we change our habits, our changing sensations indicate that this is going on. The sensations may take longer to appear as we grow older, but with patience and trust, they will appear.

THE TIME FOR IMAGING

In general, I recommend that imagery exercises be performed at the beginning of the day before breakfast, at twilight, and at the end of the day before bed. These are three potent transition points—between sleep and waking, day and night, and waking and sleep, respectively. In some instances, of course, the time of day when you perform an exercise will be related specifically to that exercise.

I want to emphasize that it is best to do imagery work before starting your daily routine—that is, before breakfast—and that you incorporate it into your waking-up and washing ritual. Imaging at this time of day is good preparation for the events and activities to come. It sets a positive attitude in facing the day ahead.

I have found that the manner in which we begin each day exerts a profound influence on how we operate and relate to people for the following twenty-four hours. Most of us have noticed that waking up from an unsettling dream can have a negative effect on our mood and behavior. We cannot resolve the issues that the dream pushed up into our consciousness. Sometimes we cannot even remember what it was that caused us to "wake up on the wrong side of the bed," and we go on to face the day grumpily, making mistakes at work, or getting into arguments. Setting a balanced mood with an imagery exercise in the morning, particularly one taken from a night dream, is helpful in determining your outlook and behavior.

THE ROAD AHEAD

The imagery exercises in the next chapter are designed to help heal a large number of maladies or disturbances, both physical and emotional.

These exercises should not be used in place of prescribed medication or instead of seeing your doctor. If you think you are ill or suffering from any of these conditions, see your doctor immediately. In addition, should your symptoms persist after practicing these imaging exercises, do not hesitate to see your doctor for a follow-up evaluation of your condition. Sometimes, you might find that your symptoms worsen slightly after beginning your imaging regimen, just as you might find that you often feel worse just before the turning point of a cold or flu. If your symptoms intensify for as long as several days up to a couple of weeks, you should not worry, but expect a breakthrough to occur shortly. If you continue to feel bad and you do not turn a corner after two weeks, consult with your doctor.

The problems the exercises deal with are arranged alphabetically. I have also provided a list that groups the entries by type of problem or bodily system. You may want to use this list to explore imagery exercises for problems related to yours.

At the beginning of each exercise, I give its name, its general intention, and the number of times it should be done. In regard to the intention of an exercise, remember it is *your* intention that counts!

I often recommend that an exercise be done in cycles of 21 days using the exercise, then 7 days off. This cycle parallels a biological rhythm that is present in all of us, most visibly in women, who are used to a cycle of three weeks of hormonal regulation and building up of body tissues and organs, followed by a week of breakdown that occurs as menstruation. Interestingly, researchers in the psychology laboratories of the University of Texas at Austin discovered that it takes 21 days to break a habit. This finding matches my clinical experience of the past fifteen years.

However, it is not etched in stone that your habit or disorder will be broken after 21 days, which is why I sometimes indicate additional cycles of imagery practice for certain more chronic ailments. Similarly, if you succeed in accomplishing your intention before the prescribed period of use, you may stop the imagery if you feel so inclined.

Your eyes should be closed for virtually all exercises. The rare exceptions are clearly identified. If closing your eyes makes you feel uncomfortable at first, keep them open. Start where you feel comfortable. (Children and young adolescents often feel more comfortable keeping their eyes open.)

In certain exercises I make no reference to breathing out. This is not an oversight. For these exercises, closing your eyes is enough. After a while you will instinctively know when there is no special breathing required for certain exercises in certain situations.

You may find yourself spontaneously modifying the exercises as you go through the imagery. Go right ahead. Let whatever comes for you come. If you find your own imagery, use it. You are calling on yourself to participate in your own healing. What you find in yourself will be most useful for your own healing.

At any point in your imagery, you might feel reluctant, anxious, or scared to go on, particularly if you come upon a situation of darkness in your imaging. If this happens, you can very easily imagine yourself bringing or finding a light of any sort to help you see your way. Your anxiety or reluctance will then evaporate.

There is no need to do a cleansing exercise before each imagery exercise. Cleansing is its own exercise and has its own purpose.

You may find that some of the exercises appear to be extremely simple techniques to deal with extremely complex problems. Remember that in imagery (as in daily life) small triggers can have large effects. Even Gordian knots can sometimes be undone swiftly. My clinical experience shows that the exercises I describe, even though they may seem simple, have the power to pierce the Gordian knots of our disorders.

In describing certain problems, I often list contributory psychological and social factors. However, I make no effort to list them all or to suggest how you might determine such factors in your own situation. Rather, I suggest that you be alert to what your imagery tells you about your life and consider how you might change the aspects of it that are associated with your disorder.

You can tape record the exercise instructions and listen to your own voice as the guide. This method can be quite powerful. Eventually, you will make up your own exercises and silently give yourself your own instructions.

You will see that a number of the exercises are variations or extensions of an exercise called **Egyptian Healing**. I call on it several times in the alphabetical listings. It can be used to help heal external bodily conditions such as skin rash, conjunctivitis, and acne, as well as for any mucous membrane surfaces and with many internal bodily troubles. You will find this exercise a powerful aid in self-healing.

Egyptian Healing

Close your eyes and breathe out three times. Then, imagine yourself standing in a large open field of green grass. See yourself stretching up toward the bright golden sun in a cloudless blue sky. See your arms becoming very long, stretching, palms up, toward the sun. The sun's rays come into your palms and circulate through the palms and fingers and beyond the fingertips so that there is a ray beyond each fingertip. If you are right-handed, at the end of each ray of the fingers of your right hand see a complete small hand. At the end of each ray of the fingers of your left hand, see an eye. There are five hands and five eyes. If you are left-handed, see the fingers on your left, the eyes on your right.

Now turn these hands and eyes toward your body and use the eyes to see your way through your body, emitting light in or on the area you are investigating so that you can see what you are doing. In the small hands you can use a golden-bristled brush for cleaning, laser-light tubes for healing, golden scalpels for surgery, cans of golden or blue-golden ointment for healing, as well as gold thread for sewing. After finishing your work, come out of your body by the same route as you went in. Any waste materials you took away with the small hands should be thrown away *behind* you. Hold your hands up toward the sun and let the small hands and eyes retract into your palms to be stored there for future use. Then open your eyes.

A final point. The following exercises are exercises in imagery. They take place in your mind reality, not in physical reality. If the exercise suggests that you use a golden-bristled brush, you of course are using this brush in your imagination. If the exercise asks you to wash your face in clear cool water, you do this in your mind, not in a sink. These exercises work with your inner subjective reality, and through this reality they change your physical reality.

CHAPTER FOUR

Blueprints for Healing:
Techniques and Effective Images for Specific Problems

You are ready to begin.

The procedure could not be simpler:

1. Sit in the Pharaoh's Posture (if the situation allows).

2. Give yourself your intention for doing the exercise. *Any intention you give yourself is correct.*

3. Close your eyes.

4. Breathe out and in the prescribed number of times. Recall that breathing out is long and slow, while breathing in is done in the normal manner. All of it is effortless.

5. Begin to do your specific imagery exercises. Let yourself receive the images effortlessly.

Work on as many ailments as you want or need to at the same time. You will find your own rhythm as you go along, especially when you find your own images. Open and close your eyes with the requisite breathing between each exercise.

Remember, everyone has the capacity to create images, to change existing imagery exercises, or to originate them. We are free to play and express ourselves in imagery. There are no restrictions, nor are there any limits to the possibilities.

Disorders Grouped by Type of Problem

Circulatory
Cardiac Arrhythmia
Cardiac Disease
Coronary Artery Disease
Edema (see under Swelling)
Hemorrhoids
Hypertension

Digestive
Anorexia
Bulimia
Gastrointestinal Disturbance
Liver Disturbance
Obesity
Pancreatitis

Emotional
Addiction
Aimlessness
Anger
Anxiety
Depression
Emotional Distress
Emotional Wounds
Ending a Relationship
Fear
Grief
Guilt
Indecisiveness
Loneliness
Obsessive Thoughts
Panic
Preparing Yourself for Surgery

Self-Doubt
Stress
Worry

Endocrine-Metabolic
Adrenal Stress
Diabetes
Thyroid Disturbance

Eyes
Cataract
Conjunctivitis
Farsightedness and Nearsightedness
Glaucoma

General
Feeling Ill
Headaches
Insomnia
Pain
Swelling (known also as Edema.
    See also Premenstrual Syndrome)

Genitourinary
Benign Tumors
Breast Cysts
Frigidity
Herpes Genitalia
Impotence
Infertility
Kidney Disturbance
Lack of Version
Polyps and Tumors

Premenstrual Syndrome
Prostate Enlargement
Vaginal Infection

Immune System
AIDS
Cancer
Chemotherapy's Debilitating
   Effects
Epstein-Barr Virus
Immune Suppression

Leukemia
Mononucleosis

Musculoskeletal
Arthritis
Bone Fracture
Muscle Spasm
Postural Disturbance
Scoliosis
Separated Shoulder
Spinal Column Problems

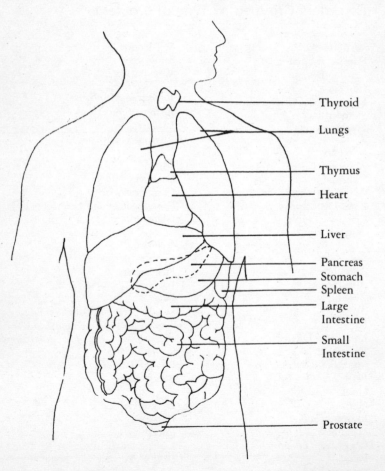

Thyroid

Lungs

Thymus

Heart

Liver

Pancreas
Stomach
Spleen
Large
Intestine

Small
Intestine

Prostate

Nervous System
Dizziness
Multiple Sclerosis

Respiratory
Asthma
Breathing Problems
Cold

Respiratory Disease
Upper Respiratory Infections

Skin
Acne
Eczema
Psoriasis
Skin Disorders
Warts

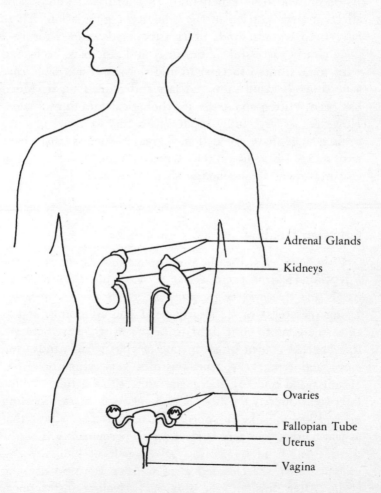

Adrenal Glands

Kidneys

Ovaries

Fallopian Tube

Uterus

Vagina

ACNE

Name: **Egyptian Healing**
Intention: To clear up acne.
Frequency: Three times a day, for 3 to 5 minutes, for three
cycles of 21 days on and 7 days off.

As those who have experienced this affliction know, acne
affects a large portion of the adolescent population. There
have been endless kinds of treatments developed for it—
none clearly successful. Vitamin A and zinc have been used
with some limited success; in addition, it is advisable that
acne sufferers avoid saturated fats and refined sugar. Much
has been written about the psychological meaning of acne.
However, so far, studies of masturbatory fantasies and re-
pressed rage have yielded no greater success than have
antibiotics. I have found that acne has to do with feelings of
embarrassment about making social contacts.

Egyptian Healing

Close your eyes, breathe out three times, and, using the
Egyptian Healing exercise (see p. 45), turn the five small
hands and five eyes to the area where the acne is located.
Using these eyes to see clearly what you are doing, and at
the same time to emit light to help you see, have a small,
fine-bristled golden brush in one of your small hands, and
clean and scrape the acne pustules very gingerly. After
cleaning and scraping the entire area, shine a tube of blue
laser light directly on the cleansed area; see the skin healing
up and looking like the normal skin around it. Know that
as you do this your acne is clearing up permanently. Use the
third small hand to apply a salve made of blue sky and
golden sun to the cleansed areas to keep the skin dry and
clean. After finishing the Egyptian Healing instructions,

raise your arms and hands toward the sun and let the rays return into your palms, where you store the small hands and the eyes. Then open your eyes.

ADDICTION

Name: **Liberating by Reexperiencing**
Intention: To find your way out of an addiction (name the addiction you have). Work on only one addiction at a time if you have more than one.
Frequency: Three times a day for up to 3 minutes for the full series, for three cycles of 21 days of use and 7 days off. If you do not have satisfactory results, use for another three cycles of 21 days on and 7 off.

We are creatures of habit. Addictions are habits carried to an extreme. They represent a loss of voluntary control over habit, to a degree that is greater than most of us ordinarily experience. Addictions are characterized by intense cravings.

Although almost everything we encounter in life can be addictive, some substances and activities seem to have more power than others to sap our will, and demonstrably are more immediately destructive. There is no need to enumerate them here, for addictive behaviors are well-known to everyone. All types of addiction can be helped by imagery.

Generally speaking, the most significant sensation or emotion associated with addictive craving is pain, mental or physical. If one's pain threshold is low, his or her addiction level tends to be high. Those who have a high pain threshold can inadvertently become addicted because an increasingly greater amount of a substance is necessary to quell their pain—a situation that can promote drug dependence.

This set of eight interrelated exercises is designed to cut addictive tendencies, and can be used along with any other addiction-recovery program in which you may be engaged. The exercises are called **Liberating by Reexperiencing,** after Arthur Janov's work described in *The Primal Scream* and other books. When you give your intention for this exercise, you should of course specify your addiction. Generally speaking, it takes 21 days to break a habit and to instill a new one. If you feel craving during the 7 days that you are not using imagery, do some "stopping exercises." Simply stop a habitual activity for a brief time—wait a moment before turning on a light switch or picking up the telephone; take another route to work; eat something different for breakfast. The more dedicated your practice of these exercises, the more profound will be the results.

Liberating by Reexperiencing

1. Close your eyes. Breathe out three times. Feel and sense yourself as a child being left cold often or for a long time. Breathe out once. Feel and sense yourself as a child being left hungry for a long time. Breathe out once. Feel and sense yourself as a child being left alone a long time. Open your eyes.

2. Close your eyes. Breathe out once. Feel and sense yourself as a child frustrated by lack of other basic needs. Open your eyes.

3. Close your eyes. Breathe out three times. Feel and live yourself as a child watching fearful confrontations. Open your eyes.

4. Close your eyes. Breathe out three times. Feel and sense what has resulted in your life from the numbing of these childhood pains. Open your eyes.

5. Close your eyes. Breathe out three times. Remove the cloak of pain. Open your eyes.

6. Close your eyes. Breathe out three times. Feel and sense that whenever there is blocked pain we also block pleasure. Open your eyes.

7. Close your eyes. Breathe out once. Feel and sense what it's like to live without repression. Open your eyes.

8. Close your eyes. Breathe out once. Sense the new quality of joy and excitement that comes from not holding back the primal pain. Open your eyes.

ADRENAL STRESS ("BURN-OUT")

Name: **Adrenal Pyramid**
Intention: To restore the body's balance; to refresh yourself.
Frequency: As needed, every hour you are awake, for 1 to 2 minutes.

When we feel overly taxed, chronically fatigued, irritable, "stressed out" or "burned out," what has happened physically is that the adrenal gland hasn't been able to keep up and is running on low. This gland, a pyramid-shaped organ sitting atop each kidney, is incredibly important for total body functioning. It produces adrenaline, the substance that wakes us up, gets us going, and stimulates our "juices." It also produces cortisone, the healing hormone known commonly as steroid, which helps the building up of tissue and muscle in the body and restores rundown tissue to health. Here's a plan for bringing vigor back to this organ—and, indeed, to any other organ. Each organ of the body has its own "brain" and can respond to your attention to it.

Adrenal Pyramid

Close your eyes and breathe out three times. Imagine yourself carrying a light, and enter your body by means of any opening you choose (pores of the skin count as openings). Find your way to the adrenal gland. Look at the gland and tell it that you love it and promise not to abuse it anymore. Then, gently caress it to show your caring. Afterward, breathe out three times, and see yourself at the top of

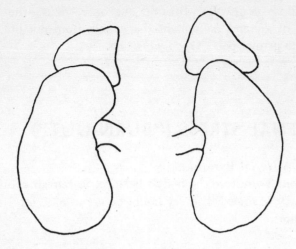

this adrenal pyramid. Now run down the steps on one side of the gland and then run up the other side, knowing that you are stimulating the gland to produce all that is necessary to keep your body in harmony. Sense the flow of hormones coming from the gland and streaming in the form of a rainbow of colors throughout the body. Now go to the other adrenal gland, breath out three times and repeat this exercise. After finishing open your eyes.

AIDS

AIDS attacks the immune system directly. (No other known disease does this.) People with AIDS have used many non-conventional treatments to help them cope with their trouble and sometimes to heal their symptoms. These treatments include imagery, meditation, prayer, diet, crystals, and healers. In one documented case, using Tibetan Buddhist meditation practice involving chanting and visualizations, a woman succeeded in reversing the positive response of her antibody blood test to negative, indicating that all AIDS virus activity had ceased.

I feel strongly that a comment on the current notion of "remission" is appropriate here. Modern medicine makes a distinction between "remission" and "cure," usually using "remission" for diseases in which there can be frequent recurrences—diseases that modern medicine generally regards as fundamentally incurable, such as AIDS. I take the position that when you are symptom-free, you are cured. In truth, virtually every disease can recur, given the proper conditions. However, in the absence of active symptoms or disease, no matter what the diagnosis, you have to be considered cured. The word *remission* actually plants in you a negative belief that the disease can or must happen again.

In my practice, each AIDS patient finds his or her own distinct path, drawing from a range of treatments, including those listed above. These self-chosen approaches all involve finding and using unique imagery exercises. The exercises are too individualized to describe here. However, the exercises that I describe in the entries for Epstein-Barr virus, herpes genitalia, and mononucleosis are excellent general ones.

AIMLESSNESS

Name: **Song of the Loom**
Intention: To give direction to your life.
Frequency: Once a day, for 3 to 5 minutes, for 3 days. Use anytime you need direction in life.

Many people suffer from a sense of purposelessness or loss of direction in life. Indeed, this feeling has become a social phenomenon. We see it in the mounting wave of homelessness throughout the world and in the large number of able-bodied people outside the labor force. (In August 1988, *The New York Times* reported that 45 percent of able-bodied New Yorkers were unemployed.) Aimlessness can be felt in small ways and to varying degrees by many of us. The following imagery exercise, based on Navajo Indian lore, will be most beneficial in correcting it.

Song of the Loom

Close your eyes. Breathe out once. See, sense, and feel yourself at your loom weaving the pattern of your life as you wish it to be. Select your threads from the myriad ones available to you. See your hands as sky and earth blending this tapestry as you hear the song the loom sings to your eternity. Then open your eyes.

ANGER

Names: **The Noose of Anger** and **Sitting Through Anger**
Intention: To relieve anger.
Frequency: Each time you experience anger; 3 minutes for the **Noose of Anger,** 1 minute for **Sitting Through Anger.**

Anger is a major stumbling block to humility. Without humility we can't be of real service to our fellow humans. Anger is a response of self-absorption and self-inflation and can lead to indifference and hatred. Where anger, indifference, and hatred reside, love cannot. Anger often gives rise to desire for revenge and sometimes its enactment. In truth, such responses only fan the flames of anger, keeping it alive. Anger, directed either at yourself or at someone else, in most instances is an overreaction to a situation. Letting it get out of control poses the dangers noted above and propels you into the position of judge and jury.

This does not mean that it is wrong or bad to experience anger. It is not a bad emotion, but one that must be managed. This applies to all emotions, positive and negative. Experience them, but don't dwell in or on them. Acknowledge their presence and then deal with them.

The antidote to anger is forgiveness. Forgiveness is first directed at yourself and then at the one toward whom you are angry.

When you feel anger, begin the inner process called "confession of the heart" (after Philo, the first-century Western philosopher), in which you acknowledge your error of getting angry and ask yourself for forgiveness. (If you are religiously or spiritually inclined, you can ask God for forgiveness.) Afterward, begin the outer process of asking the one toward whom your anger was directed for forgiveness (called "confession of the lips"). Apology is one such form of asking for forgiveness.

Here are two imagery exercises for handling anger. Please note that the root of the word *anger* means "constricting."

The Noose of Anger

Close your eyes. Breathe out three times. Remove the noose that is constricting you. At each knot—a noose has up to thirteen knots—see what is creating your anger and correct it. Don't allow yourself to mix in other emotions in this exercise; concentrate on anger alone. After finishing all the knots, open your eyes, knowing that the anger is gone.

Sitting Through Anger

Close your eyes. Breathe out three times. See yourself sitting inside your anger. Find your way out and look at it. Decide what you want to do with it, and do it. Transform it, dispose of it—it's your choice. Breathe out once, and after ridding yourself of anger, place in the newly vacated space an opposite image, such as sitting in the center of a rose, or floating on a cloud. Remember, it's best to find your own images, the ones coming directly from your own experience. Then open your eyes, knowing that the anger is gone.

ANOREXIA

Name: **The New Birth**
Intention: To reconnect to eating.
Frequency: Each time you consider eating, for 1 to 2 minutes, as needed.

Like bulimia, anorexia (*an* = without; *rexia* = longing for) is a disorder connected with conflicts having to do with growing up, more specifically with entering adolescence. The anorectic person refuses to take the step into adolescence, the bulimic person flirts with taking the step. An anorectic who risks dying by refusing to eat, or who wants to die, can in fact die if her weight falls below a critical level. I say "her" because the overwhelming number of anorectics are female.

If you are an anorectic, the following may help you.

The New Birth

Close your eyes and breathe out three times. See, sense, feel, and know yourself as you were before you were born. Be comfortable and contented. Breathe out once and see yourself head-down at the entrance to the birth canal and experience the process of birth. After being born, breathe out once and see yourself being placed at your mother's breast by your father. Know that you are worthy of being nourished by them, and as a baby forgive them for any hurts they may have inflicted. Breathe out once and see, sense, and feel yourself being satisfyingly nourished at your mother's breast, knowing that you are going to grow straight to become the ruler of yourself. Then open your eyes.

ANXIETY

Names: **Breathing, Desert Storm, American Indian, Blue Light, Colored Spiral Maze, The Mummy, and Calm Water**

Intention: To put the lid on anxiety when it occurs.

Frequency: Daily, as needed. Do any exercise, or a combination of the exercises, whenever you experience anxiety, for up to 3 minutes each.

Along with depression, this most ubiquitous of negative emotional states is generated from within—as opposed to fear, which is a response to something happening outside of us. The literal meaning of *anxiety* is "twisted rope"! Anxiety is *always* produced in relation to time—that is, in regard to concerns about the future. We cannot actually know the future; it is *only* potential, not something that actually exists. However, we tend to treat the future as an actual thing, susceptible to being manipulated, controlled, or modified. This unfortunate self-deception, from which most of us suffer, prompts the fretting and discomfort that characterize anxiety. It is unlikely that any of us will elude this trap entirely. At one time or another, we will feel anxious. Here are seven exercises that will help you get quickly through your moments of anxiety. Some may suit you more than others. Select the one(s) that bring you relief.

Breathing

Bring your attention immediately to your breathing. Breathing is *always* altered when we are anxious. Controlled breathing brings control of anxiety. Start to let out long, slow exhalations through your mouth, and take in *normal*— not exaggerated—inhalations through your nose. Continue to do this until you feel quiet. *Do not* take in big, deep inhalations, as this will increase your anxiety and may make you feel faint.

Desert Storm

Close your eyes and breathe out three times. See yourself entering a desert carrying a backpack. As you walk, you notice darkness looming ahead of you. You know this means that a sandstorm of anxiety is coming toward you. As it approaches, see yourself removing a folded tent from your backpack. Unfold it and set it up, driving the four pegs into place, raising the tent, then going in through the flap and closing it behind you. Sit peacefully in your tent as you hear the sand blowing around and over the tent. Know that when you hear the sandstorm pass completely, your anxiety has passed. Then open your eyes.

American Indian

Close your eyes and breathe out three times. See yourself at the seashore. The sky is clear. See and feel your anxiety abiding in you like a stone or rock. Let the water and wind erode this rock, washing and blowing away the particles that remain after the erosion. Know that when all the particles have gone, your anxiety has gone as well. Then open your eyes.

Blue Light

Close your eyes, breathe out three times, and see yourself entering a beautiful meadow. See yourself taking in the blue-golden light, a mixture of bright golden sun and cloudless blue sky, and breathing out the carbon dioxide as gray smoke, which you watch drift away and disappear. Let the blue light circulate through your bloodstream, reaching everywhere in your being, helping you to become calm and quiet. Let the blue light circulate through your fingertips and beyond, to encircle your body in a sapphire blue glow. See the inner and outer blue light linking. Know that your body is a bridge allowing this linking. When you see the blue light link, know that your anxiety has passed. Open your eyes.

Colored Spiral Maze

Close your eyes, breathe out three times, and see yourself going through a colored spiral maze. When you exit the maze, know that your anxiety has gone, and open your eyes.

The Mummy

Close your eyes, breathe out three times, and see yourself as a mummy wrapped in bandages. Remove the bandages, roll them into a ball, and throw it away. Breathe out once and find a cave. Go deep into it and find your own sarcophagus (mummy tomb). Go into the coffin and lie there, again as a mummy wrapped in bandages. Remove the bandages, knowing that your anxiety has left you. Then leave the coffin, come out of the cave, see the blue sky, and open your eyes.

Calm Water

Close your eyes. Breathe out three times. See and sense your entire being becoming like the surface of calm water reflecting the starry sky. When you have fully sensed this, know that your anxiety has gone, and open your eyes.

ARTHRITIS

Name: **The Octopus** and **The Tide**
Intention: To shrink the nodules and/or to heal arthritis.
Frequency: These exercises can be done together. Do **The Octopus** as needed, for 30 seconds. Do **The Tide** 3 times a day, for three cycles of 21 days of use, followed by 7 days off. In the first week, the duration of the exercise should be 2 to 3 minutes; in the second and third weeks, 1 to 2 minutes. After you complete three cycles, evaluate your condition. If you require more work, apply another three cycles of 21 days on and 7 off. If necessary, repeat again for another three cycles.

Arthritis is an immobilizing illness limiting our range of motion and thus impairing our freedom on many levels. It expresses a simultaneous dysfunction of motion, movement, and freedom in our physical, emotional, and social lives. Suppressed anger has often been associated with arthritis, and my clinical experience has borne this out. Anger often requires a physical outlet through the muscles and joints in order to express itself. If these outlets are lacking, then tension is created in the joints and muscles, creating a new habit of holding back. I have found the following imagery exercises to be of inestimable value in treating this condition. They are called **The Octopus** and **The Tide**.

Please note that the more sensory awareness you experience in the affected area during these exercises, the more success you will have. We all have different levels of awareness and patience. Take heart, be perseverant. If you are diligent, sensory awareness will come. Remember, you don't have to strive to sense something; in fact, the more you strive, the less you'll sense. Just do your job and *wait* for your body's response.

The Octopus

Close your eyes. Breathe out three times. See your arms (or legs, or fingers, or toes) as octopus tentacles, sinewy and undulating, elongating out in front of you for at least a mile. See and sense the flexibility of these members elongating freely, allowing you to bend them in all directions. Then open your eyes.

The Tide

Close your eyes and breathe out three times. See yourself at a beautiful beach, a familiar place that you have visited or seen before. The sand is golden, the sky cloudless blue, and the sun bright and golden. Find the place on the beach where the sand and water meet. Lie down on your back at that point, with the soles of your feet toward the water, and cover yourself with wet sand, leaving exposed only the soles of your feet, your face, and your head. The sand-and-water mixture acts as a pumice compound, cleansing your skin. See the tide coming in very quickly, entering the soles of your feet. Sense spiral currents of water washing away all the accumulations of waste products there, dissolving any deposits and eliminating toxins. The tide then begins to go out, and the current reverses, flowing out of your feet slowly. See the waste products emerging as black or gray strands being carried away on the outgoing tide.

The tide comes back in quickly and again enters through the soles, then moves up into your feet and ankles, washing away all the waste products and toxins there. As the tide goes out, the spiral current again reverses. Sense it flowing from your ankles, through your feet, and down into the soles of your feet as black or gray strands, which are carried away by the outgoing tide. The sand-and-water compound thoroughly cleanses the outside of your feet and ankles.

Once again the tide comes back very quickly through the soles of your feet, the spiral current now passing into your feet and ankles and up into your legs and knees, washing away all the waste and toxins there. Sense the spiral current massaging the muscles, helping the ligaments and tendons to stretch, and cleaning the cartilage and kneecaps until they are gleaming white. As the tide starts going out, sense the spiral current reversing, flowing back down slowly through your legs and calves, slowly into your ankles, your feet, and out through your soles. See the wastes emerge as black or gray strands being carried away in the outgoing tide, the pumice compound having thoroughly cleansed the outside of your knees.

The tide comes back quickly now through your soles, the spiral current going through your feet, ankles, legs, knees, and thighs, through the groin and into the lower abdomen and spinal column, through the abdomen, into the chest cavity and upper spinal column, into the neck and cervical vertebrae, and through the shoulders. Sense the current going down through the upper arms, into the elbows, and down the forearms into the wrists, cleaning out all the toxins, washing away all the wastes, eroding all the accumulations, massaging the bones, ligaments, tendons, and muscles, making them all gleaming white and seeing them stretching and elongating. The tide reverses again and goes out. The spiral current reverses and goes back slowly from the wrists up through the forearms. Sense it returning through the elbows, upper arms, shoulders, neck, into the chest cavity, down into the abdominal cavity, through the groin, thighs, knees, legs, ankles, and feet, and see the waste products coming out through the soles as black or gray strands and being carried away by the outgoing tide. This reverse process is to be done *slowly* in contrast to the incoming tide and spirals, which come in *quickly*.

See the nodules disappearing as the current cleans them out. Then stand up, dive into the ocean, and swim out to the horizon. See your arms and legs becoming immensely long, and then your torso becoming long as well. Your limbs are to move freely as you swim freestyle. As you reach the horizon, turn over on your back and swim to shore, using a backstroke as your limbs again become immensely long and freely flowing and your torso becomes elongated as well. When you reach the shore, come out of the water and let the sun dry you. Then find a light gown or robe on the ground near you, and put it on before coming back to the chair in which you are sitting, breathing out, and opening your eyes.

Be patient with these exercises. Reduction of nodules takes time. Thankfully, this is not an immediately life-threatening illness, so you have the luxury of a relatively anxiety-free waiting period while you work on this ailment.

ASTHMA

Name: **Exorcism**
Intention: To heal the lungs.
Frequency: Daily (in the morning), for 3 minutes (1 minute anytime you experience wheezing), for 7 days.

Name: **Pine Forest**
Intention: To stem an asthmatic attack.
Frequency: At the onset of an attack, for 3 to 5 minutes.

Name: **Light in the Lake**
Intention: To breathe normally.
Frequency: As needed, every 15 to 30 minutes, for 2 to 3 minutes.

Asthma is a respiratory ailment characterized by wheezing on exhalation. It affects lung resiliency, so that over time the lung tissue loses its capacity to stretch, ultimately leading to serious breathing difficulties that may even result in death. Allergy, infection, and emotions contribute to the development of asthma. Allergy is a response to certain

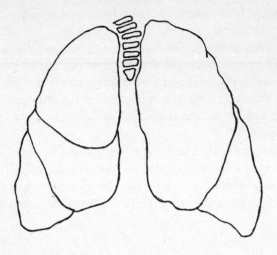

environmental substances, while infection is associated with bacterial invasion. The emotional contribution seems to come mainly from knotted dependency problems, particularly related to struggles for independence from maternal influence, although sometimes the distressing influence can be paternal. Either way, however, my clinical experience has shown that the issue is almost always related to a parent. The asthmatic wheeze has a positive as well as a negative meaning. The positive meaning is expression of wanting to breathe freely—to become free. The negative meaning is generally considered to bespeak the fear of breaking loose from parental influence.

Regarding the first exercise, **Exorcism**, do not be concerned that it might produce guilt or pain. This imagery is not a guilt-provoking process, nor is it dangerous.

Exorcism

Close your eyes. Breathe out three times. See yourself taking off your clothes. See yourself in a mirror nude from the neck down. In the mirror, with your right forefinger (left forefinger if you are left-handed) touch on and into your upper chest area from the front all the way around to the back, making a complete circle. Now touch the area of greatest discomfort and *see to whom you can't breathe—that is, see whose face appears in the area*. Who is restricting your breathing, and what color appears there? Breathe that color out via long, slow exhalations while removing from the area whomever you've seen, at first as gently as you can. If the person does not leave easily, use increasing force, going from the gentle to the vigorous, perhaps eventually going so far as to use a golden scalpel to cut out the person. As you are removing this person, tell him/her that he/she is no longer permitted to stay in your body, that he/she has to leave and to stay at a far distance from your body; that he/she will no longer be welcome in your body and will never be allowed to enter your body again. After the removal, see yourself becoming very, very tall and reaching your arms far up into the sky, all the way to the sun. Take a piece of the sun in your palms and place it in the space just vacated. See the area healing, and see how you look and feel. Then, put your clothes back on, breathe out once, and open your eyes, knowing that you are breathing easily.

Pine Forest

Close your eyes. Breathe out three times and see yourself in a pine forest. Stand next to a pine tree and breathe in the aromatic fragrance of the pine. As you breathe out, sense this exhalation traveling down through your body and going out through the soles of your feet; see the breath exiting as gray smoke and being buried deep in the earth. Then open your eyes, breathing easily.

Light in the Lake

Close your eyes, breathe out three times, and go to the bottom of a lake, breathing in easily and exhaling slowly as you enter the lake and go under water. Sit on the lake bottom quietly enveloped by golden light. Afterward, leave the lake and sit under a maple tree near the lake. Take a maple leaf, touch it, and experience its texture. Then enter into the leaf and become one with the breathing process of the leaf. Next, leave the leaf, knowing that your breathing is regulated. Open your eyes.

BENIGN TUMORS (see Polyps and Tumors)

BONE FRACTURE

Name: **Weaving the Marrow**
Intention: To heal a fracture.
Frequency: Every 3 to 4 hours while awake, for 3 minutes.
  Significant results should be seen in one to two weeks.

Name: **Feeding the Bone**
Intention: To heal a fracture.
Frequency: Every 3 to 4 hours while awake, for 3 minutes.
  Look for results in one to two weeks.

The following exercises are extremely effective in helping to heal simple bone fractures. Look into the emotional and social circumstances surrounding you when the break occurred. As I described earlier, a friend broke her wrist bone. It so happened that the break occurred while she was en route to a meeting at which she was going to announce a "break" with the organization for which she worked. A similar situation occurred with another patient who was going to announce a "breakup" with a girlfriend. He was on his way to meet her, slipped, and fractured a leg bone.

A break in a bone is often connected to a change of direction in life. To heal quickly, you must be willing to accept that the fracture is a consequence of changing a very familiar life pattern. As with all imagery work, you must be aware that the body is speaking to you about change.

My bone-fracture patients experience a greater sense of "coming together" (healing) rapidly once they discover the relationship between their physical and experiential "breaks."

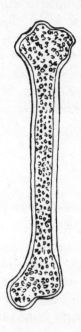

Weaving the Marrow

Close your eyes, breathe out three times, and see the ends of the broken bone as they look now. See the two ends placed together. Breathe out once. See and sense the marrow flowing from one end into the other. See this white marrow carried in channels of blue light flowing through the red bloodstream, seeing the materials flowing back and forth between the two ends, forming a woven net that brings the two ends close. See the two ends knitting together perfectly until you can no longer see any sign of a break. Know that the bone is now one, and then open your eyes.

Feeding the Bone

Close your eyes and breathe out three times. See your broken bone as it now looks. See the two ends placed together. See and sense the marrow flowing from one end into the other. Then see yourself eating radishes. See the calcium and magnesium from the radishes being carried as particles into the bone, aiding the healing. See the bone elongating as the ends knit together. Then open your eyes.

BREAST CYSTS (see also Polyps and Tumors)

Name: **The Chimes of Life**
Intention: To eliminate breast cysts.
Frequency: Three times a day (early morning, twilight, bedtime), for 3 to 5 minutes, for 21 days. If the cyst has not disappeared, wait 7 days and do another two cycles of 21 days of imagery with 7 days off in between.

This common finding in women has eluded a consistently successful treatment. Certainly it would be valuable to look at the emotional/social issues connected with it. Frustration at not being able to nurture or be nurtured in a given relationship is one example. (Research also suggests that diet may be involved in breast cysts. Caffeine, cola, and chocolate may all contribute to them; vitamin E and lysine, an amino acid, may help reduce them.) "Ann," a patient who successfully used **The Chimes of Life** exercise—her cysts were gone when she had her last checkup—reported: "Each time I hear a chime sound, or uplifting music of any kind, I immediately respond to it by allowing it to move through my breasts and let it act as a resonant healing power. I keep seeing the cysts getting smaller, breaking up, and disappearing. I see my breasts as free of blockages and full of blue-white light."

The Chimes of Life

Close your eyes and breathe out three times. See yourself wearing a jeweled breastplate. It is translucent, and each jewel is a chime with its own beautiful tone. As you tap each chime *lightly* with the tip of your forefinger, hear the melody of the chimes becoming stronger and becoming a healing melody. Feel the sound resonating in your breasts: the tissues respond, as do the cells. See and feel the impurities shaken free, the cyst(s) breaking up as this sound separates the pure from the impure. As this happens, see blue-golden light circulating through the area, these rays discharging an energy that courses through you. See and hear this sound and light becoming a shower of movement in your breasts, dispelling the dark impurities and carrying them down through the body and out through the soles of your feet: see the cyst(s) disappear with the impurities. Then open your eyes.

BREATHING PROBLEMS
(see also **Respiratory Disease**)

Name: **Threading the Needle**
Intention: To achieve normal breathing.
Frequency: As needed, four times a day, 1 to 2 minutes for
   each of the exercises.

It has been amazing to find in my clinical experience how much emotional trouble—like anxiety—is intimately connected to breathing disturbances. Many of these disturbances are so subtle that we are unaware that a problem exists. You can have a slightly deviated nasal septum, or you may have naturally narrow nostrils, preventing the inflow of oxygen. The less oxygen you are able to take in, the more anxious you are likely to become. We know that breathing changes when we experience different emotional states such as fear, anger, and anxiety. There is also a different pattern of breathing when we are deeply concentrated on some task or are reading. Breath is life. As such, it is the physical equivalent of faith. Faith and living are analogous. When there are breathing problems, there is a break in living and in faith as well. While we breathe we are alive. It is our main source of energy and our regulator of self-confidence. Learning to breathe properly can do much to restore balance and a sense of equilibrium when it is needed quickly. Following is a set of breathing exercises. Use any one or any combination of them that you find helpful.

Threading the Needle

1. Close your eyes and become conscious of your breathing, and know that as you do you are ridding yourself of hindering influences and are feeling liberated. Open your eyes.

2. Close your eyes. Breathe out three times. See and feel how you don't have to correct your breathing pattern all at once, but that you can use it as a starting point, even if it is a faulty one. Then open your eyes.

3. Close your eyes. Breathe out three times. See and feel the inner movement of your natural breathing until the breath, left to itself, returns to its normal pattern. Stay with this rhythm a long moment, then open your eyes.

4. Close your eyes and breathe out three times. Feel and

sense an emotional state. See it and be aware of how your breathing is changing. Open your eyes.

5. Close your eyes and breathe out once. Feel and see how negative feelings reduce our breathing. What happens? Then open your eyes.

6. Close your eyes and breathe out three times. Sense and hear how, when we sigh, we are relieved. Sense and feel how, when you are at peace, you are breathing more with the diaphragm. Then open your eyes.

BULIMIA (binge eating and purging)

Name: **The Milky Way**
Intention: To curb compulsive eating.
Frequency: Before indulging in eating, until you feel a
   sense of fullness in the abdomen.

Bulimia is a semitechnical term for overeating, or bingeing, followed by vomiting. The bulimic can eat great quantities yet remain thin, due to vomiting. Generally, this disturbed eating pattern concerns the emergence of inhibitions about growing up. This difficulty affects females primarily and speaks to what happens to them in early puberty, when the sexual and emotional changes taking place are not honored by their fathers, who are made anxious by the budding womanhood of their daughters. In response to the trouble in her father, the young adolescent girl punishes her own body and mind as she responds strongly to her father's problem. To get well, and not just end her bulimia, she needs to shed unnecessary guilt feelings and assume her adult female status. Here we work on the immediate problem—curbing the gluttonous eating. Relief from this problem is likely to bring new self-understanding that will guide the bulimic in taking additional steps in self-healing. I use an exercise derived from the root meaning of *bulimia,* which is "cow."

Use this exercise, in which you envision the vastness of our galaxy, before you are about to indulge. If you sense the fullness in your abdomen, you have made good headway. It takes faith to allow yourself to take this step, and trust that a nurturing environment will develop around you. If you take the step, the universe will provide that environment.

The Milky Way

Close your eyes. Breathe out three times and see a cow grazing contentedly in a meadow. After she finishes, see her jumping over the Milky Way. See this Milky Way streaming from the cow's udder down to you as you stand under the moon with face up toward the milky flow, letting it flow into your open mouth. Feel satiated and satisfied. Then sense your fullness, and open your eyes.

CANCER

Name: **God's Hands** and **Lightning Hands**
Intention: To clean out cancer.
Frequency: Three times a day, for 1 to 2 minutes, for nine cycles of 21 days of use and 7 days off.

Cancer is a disease fed by many sources: emotional (loss, grief, depression); environmental (environmental contamination of water, air, food, and the effects of radiation exposure); social (breakdowns in our social, familial, or business relationships); moral/ethical (errors in the integrity of our moral behavior). Becoming aware of these contributory elements is an extremely valuable step in promoting cancer healing. If you feel stymied in working these matters out for yourself, seek the help of a trained clinician who is accepting of these conditions as contributory factors in cancer. Don't feel any compunctions about seeking this help, and, above all, do not feel guilty or intimidated if your physician does not agree with your decision to explore additional therapies. Do what *you* need to do. Your life comes first and foremost. Take the authority for yourself.

Here are two general cancer-healing exercises that can be employed by anyone suffering from this disease. I cannot prescribe specific cancer exercises because cancer-healing through imagery *must* be monitored by the practitioner. I mentioned earlier that imagery is associated with strong physiological activity—in one sense, that is what this book is about—and we must be careful *not* to move cancer cells by imagery activity. The dose and intensity of the imagery must be adjusted to each case individually. However, the general exercises given here can be useful in ameliorating the overall condition. The first exercise is for those who have religious inclinations.

God's Hands

Close your eyes. Breathe out three times and see yourself as *being* God's hands. Breathe out once. Seeing your hands as the Almighty's, touch the place on and in the diseased area, gently cleaning out all the dirt and contamination and then *putting* in order what has been in disorder (for example, weaving together the fibers of the wall of the colon). Then, breathe out once and see your body in *perfect* condition. Your face is happy and smiling and your brain is working in the most adequate way. Like yourself, and see yourself being washed by a light sunshower coming from above. Be proud of the body you have constructed. Then open your eyes.

Lightning Hands

Close your eyes. Breathe out three times and see your hands become lightning bolts. Enter your body with them to the place of disease. Take out what is there as you inhale quickly, then quickly remove the lightning hands, bringing the diseased matter with them. Throw it all behind you. Then see a small waterfall above you and bathe in it, feeling thoroughly cleansed. Then open your eyes.

CARDIAC ARRHYTHMIA

Names: **Crystal Heart, Musical Triangle,** and **Flower Petals**
Intention: To make your heartbeat regular.
Frequency: Daily, as needed, each time you are aware of irregular heartbeat, till you sense a regular heartbeat.

Irregularities of heartbeat are commonplace in our culture. They are generally discovered in the course of a physical exam by a doctor. Many of the irregularities are considered "normal" in that they don't reflect any active heart disease, although you may feel discomfort from the irregular beat.

"Mary," a 50-year-old woman, summoned me to her hospital room where she had just been admitted suffering from severe cardiac arrhythmia. Her husband had died suddenly some months before. She was deeply in love with this man and her heart was responding to the shock of this loss. When I saw her I found her hooked up to a cardiac monitor that was being watched at the nurses' station some distance from her room. I closed the door to her room to ensure privacy and she told the nurses that she did not want to be interrupted for the next 30 minutes. She then did the **Musical Triangle** exercise, described below, at the end of which the nurse on duty came bursting through the door, shouting to see if Mary was all right. We were both stunned at first, but Mary pulled herself together and demanded to know what the nurse was doing there. The nurse said that she had been watching the cardiac monitor screen at the nurses' station and had seen the electrocardiogram signal become *normal*. Thinking that something must be wrong with Mary because of the sudden change in the cardiogram, she had rushed to the room to check. Mary was released from the hospital shortly afterward. She continued the imagery and her health remained stable.

Please be aware that most arrhythmia, like palpitations (the experience of sensing the heart beating against the chest wall), has a significant emotional component. Anxiety is one emotion commonly connected with arrhythmia; grief is another. Arrhythmia should not be treated as strictly a physical problem.

Here are a few imagery exercises to bring about a regular heartbeat.

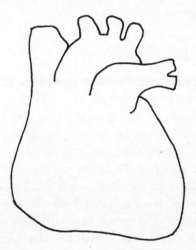

Crystal Heart

Close your eyes. Breathe out three times and see your heart as a crystal. Clean all the dark spots from it by any means of cleansing that feels comfortable to you. Let a shower of light come from above, cleaning the crystal heart. Then see the heart fill with fluid and become translucent, and as the fluid leaves, see the heart become transparent. See, sense, and feel this change from translucency to transparency until the heart quiets. Then open your eyes.

Musical Triangle

Close your eyes. Breathe out three times and see a musical triangle that you place in the center of your heart. Each of the three sides is golden. The three curves of the angles where the sides join are different colors: one red, one blue, one yellow. With a soft golden mallet, play each of the three sides, hearing a harmonious sound, knowing that as you play, your heart is quieting down. When the sound is completely harmonious, your heart will be in tempo. Then open your eyes.

Flower Petals

Close your eyes. Breathe out three times. It is dawn and the sun is rising on your heart, which is shaped like a flower. The sunlight enters the flower, and the petals begin to open very delicately as the process of life and circulation of life fill it through the stem and down to the roots. Now feel the sap coming up from the depths of the earth, going through the stem of the flower and filling every petal until the entire flower is open. Presently, it becomes dusk and the sun is setting; the petals begin to close as the sun goes down so that the flower closes for the night. Then open your eyes.

CARDIAC DISEASE

Names: **The Arrows of Hurt, The Cosmic Heart,** and
Gateway to Heaven
Intention: To heal the heart and relieve heartache.
Frequency: Twice a day, for 3 minutes, for cycles of 21 days
on and 7 days off until the heart returns to normal.

Simply put, the heart is the seat of love. Cardiac arrhythmia
(p. 76), coronary artery disease (p. 85), and heart attack
all involve trouble regarding love. Being heartsick, having
heartache, eating your heart out, all have their roots in the
arena of love. We can be spurned, jilted, disappointed,
divorced, heartbroken, and our hearts reflect these situations. I have found that becoming aware of this connection
brings relief and helps the healing process. It's amazing how
awareness of the connections between physical and emotional processes can direct the flow from illness to well-
being. In every case that I have treated, I have found that
using mental imagery has not only yielded insight into the
love–heart-disease connection, but that it has speeded up the

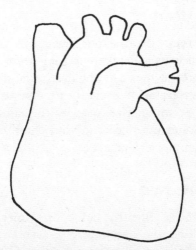

healing process as well. One example is the man I described in chapter 2, whose heart problems were intimately associated with his feeling that his wife did not love him.

Cardiac disease is a diagnosis made by an M.D. If you have cardiac disease, these exercises should be useful. Choose the exercise you want and use it for yourself each day until your heart returns to normal. You can vary the exercises, if you want. While doing any exercise, look also at your disappointment or sadness about love, your grief, or whatever, and acknowledge it; even tell someone about it. Try not to keep it in.

The Arrows of Hurt

Close your eyes. Breathe out three times. Unzip your chest wall. Reach in and take out your heart. Remove all the arrows of hurt and toss them away. Clean up all the sore spots where the arrows were. Gently massage the heart, replace it back in your chest, and rezip your chest wall. Listen to your heartbeat and sense and feel the now strengthened heart muscle becoming alive. Open your eyes.

The Cosmic Heart

Close your eyes. Breathe out three times. Unzip your chest wall. Reach in and take out your heart. Clean it and massage it gently. Now, toss the heart straight up into the cosmos and retrieve it. See the heart now as clear crystal reflecting as a prism all the colors of the rainbow. Replace this now clean and pure heart in your chest and rezip your chest wall. Then open your eyes.

Gateway to Heaven

Close your eyes. Breathe out three times. Enter your heart. There, find the gateway to heaven. See what happens. Sense and feel your heart responding. Open your eyes.

CATARACT

Name: **The Waterfall**
Intention: To heal a cataract.
Frequency: Every 1 to 2 hours while awake, for 3 minutes, for three cycles of 21 days of use with 7 days off in between. If needed, repeat for another three cycles of 21 days on, 7 days off.

A cataract is an opacity of the lens of the eye created by deposits of calcium in the lens. Consequently, vision eventually becomes blurred to the point of blindness. Naturally, we would look not only for physical reasons for this difficulty but also for emotional ones. My experience has demonstrated that each person suffering from a cataract did not want to see something that was especially wrenching emotionally. One man, for instance, literally did not want to see himself growing old.

New surgical techniques for cataracts seem effective. But recurrences are frequent. As cataracts are slow growing you might want to try this exercise before resorting to surgery.

For purposes of our imagery work, it is useful to know that a cataract is also a waterfall. This image is immensely valuable in framing imagery that can be used to clear up the opacity.

Try to be relaxed when doing this exercise. Do not make the mistake of becoming impatient for a miracle. It took a number of years to arrive at this condition, and it may not disappear overnight. As I stated earlier, healing requires active participation on your part and happens over time.

One other note: You may at first be surprised by an image that refers to a paste of saliva. In the miracle performed by Jesus when he helped a blind man see, he spit into the blind man's eyes. This form of healing was commonly used by the prophets of the Holy Land.

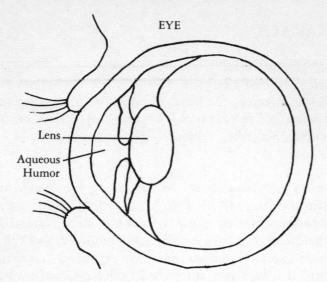

EYE

Lens

Aqueous
Humor

The Waterfall

Close your eyes. Breathe out three times and find yourself
standing under a large waterfall. Imagine that you can
remove the lens from your eye and see it in your hand. See
it cloudy, and put it under the water and wash it thoroughly in rushing, clean, clear, scouring water. See and
sense the cataract eroding until all the particles are washed
away. Breathe out once. Before replacing the lens in your
eye, have a great holy man (if you are religious) or someone
you love dearly place a paste of saliva onto the lens and into
the empty space where the lens was, to keep the space free
of further deposits. Then replace the lens. Know that it has
cleared up. Open your eyes.

CHEMOTHERAPY'S DEBILITATING EFFECTS

Name: **River of Sunlight**
Intention: To make chemotherapy a friend.
Frequency: Each morning, for 1 to 2 minutes, in the 7 days
    prior to receiving chemotherapy.

Chemotherapy is the treatment offered to most cancer patients either in conjunction with or instead of surgery. The
chemical agents used are extremely toxic and almost invariably produce debilitating effects that are a natural consequence of the drugs' activity.* Chemotherapy can also sap
the will, and it is usually extremely difficult for a person
undergoing chemotherapy to maintain the attention required for effective imagery work. However, the following
exercise is helpful in offsetting the weakening produced by
these anticancer agents.

River of Sunlight

Close your eyes. Breathe out three times and see the
chemicals coming into your body as rivers of sunlight flowing throughout, flushing out the cancer cells and destroying
them. Know that these chemicals are medicine that is
helping you to heal as the tumor is weakened, shrunken,
and destroyed. It is a friend that has come to help you.
Then open your eyes.

---

*These debilitating effects are often called side effects. But there is no
such thing as a side effect of a drug. Every drug has its effect. There are
no independent or side actions of a drug. It does what it does. If it
produces damage to the body while removing something injurious, then
that is what it does.

COLDS (see Upper Respiratory Infections)

CONJUNCTIVITIS

Name: **Egyptian Healing**
Intention: To clear up inflammation.
Frequency: Three times a day, for 1 to 2 minutes, for 21 days.

This inflammation of the mucous membrane of the eyelid, usually the lower one, creates a redness and swelling of the area. It is a benign condition and can reflect a number of factors that include tiredness and fatigue, vitamin deficiency—especially vitamin C—and crying connected with a sense of loss and grief. This last factor should be considered as highly contributory to eye inflammation.

Regardless of the predisposing factor or factors, the exercise described on page 82 or the **Egyptian Healing** exercise presented here can be quite beneficial.

Egyptian Healing

Close your eyes. Breathe out three times. See yourself in a large open field and proceed to use the **Egyptian Healing** process. Turning your eyes and small hands to your eyelid(s), see how the eyelid(s) looks using your five eyes, and then use them to see clearly everything your small hands are doing. In one of your small hands have a golden feather with which you clean out all the redness and inflammation from the conjunctiva. With another of your small hands lay a line of blue laser light from a laser tube along the track of the conjunctiva where you have just cleaned away the redness. See, sense, and know that the conjunctiva is healing normally. Afterward, finish off the **Egyptian Healing** process in the usual way described for this exercise (see p. 45). Then, breathe out and open your eyes.

CORONARY ARTERY DISEASE

Name: **White Snow**
Intention: To open clogged arteries.
Frequency: Every hour while awake, for 1 to 2 minutes, for cycles of 21 days on and 7 days off until the arteries have opened.

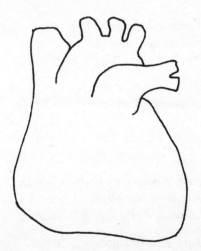

Troubles with the heart, as I explained earlier under *Cardiac Disease,* always involve troubles with love. Keep this in mind while doing this exercise. Try to see the disappointment or sadness in love from which you are suffering.

White Snow

Close your eyes. Breathe out three times. Look into a mirror and see the ugly, craggy electrocardiogram as a bilious green color. In the mirror see it turn into a sunny horizon of pure white snow with a straight, sure, shiny black line stretched from one end to the other. See the line as comprised of black, healthy poppy seeds. Know that your arteries are opening. Then open your eyes.

DEPRESSION

Name: **The Drop of Hope**
Intention: To wash out despair.
Frequency: Three times a day, 1 to 3 minutes, for 21 days.

Name: **The Staircase of Life**
Intention: To overcome obsessive thinking connected with depression.
Frequency: Every 2 hours but not more than six times per day, for 2 to 3 minutes, until you find relief.

Name: **Blowing Away the Dark Clouds**
Intention: To stop being blue.
Frequency: As needed, for up to 1 minute.

Name: **Crossing the Bridge**
Intention: To rid yourself of regret.
Frequency: Twice a day, for 2 to 3 minutes, for 21 days.

Name: **Rebury the Dead**
Intention: To clear up excessive mourning of a dead loved one.
Frequency: Once a day, for 2 to 3 minutes, for 7 days.
Names: **Clean a Space, Fingerpainting,** and **Spiral of Energy**

Intention: To regain depleted energy, or to give yourself new energy.

Frequency: Three times a day, for 2 to 3 minutes, for cycles of 21 days of use and 7 days off until energy is restored.

Name: **Sailing Out of the Doldrums**
Intention: To get out of the doldrums.
Frequency: Two to three times a day, for 1 minute, for up to 21 days until the state is passed.

Name: **Out of Limbo**
Intention: To overcome depression connected with feeling stuck.
Frequency: Three times a day, for 1 to 2 minutes, for 21 days.

Name: **Swallowing the Rainbow**
Intention: To overcome depression connected with feelings of hopelessness or isolation or internal mood shifts not connected to outside circumstances.
Frequency: Four times a day, for 1 minute, for 21 days.

Depression in its various forms—grief, mourning, melancholy, sadness, brooding, moodiness, and the like—is clearly the world's most ubiquitously experienced chronic emotional disorder. In a large number of cases, these various forms are directly related to *loss* and/or to self-directed anger. Most of us lose something every day—a person, an ideal, a thing, a plan, a dream of success, a hope. Depending on the degree and intensity of the loss, many of us react with one of the states mentioned above—such as grief or mourning. If this state persists for an inordinately long time (certainly more than three months) and functioning begins to diminish, along with appetite, sleep, interest in life, and sexual drive, then we are facing full-blown depression. There are a great many other tendencies or symptoms that we might see expressed. This is why I present here a varied array of exercises. You are likely to find one or more of them useful.

The ubiquity of depressed states underscores the universality of loss. Almost no one is exempt from the experience of depression. It is the forerunner of dying and death and requires our utmost attention and concern. From my point of view, nothing on earth demands our attention more, since at some point everyone has this experience. Paradoxically, this universal experience has to be met with equanimity, not with consternation. Loss, as it affects us all, represents the continual chance for us to come to terms with the frailty of physical life.

The Drop of Hope (two exercises)

1. Close your eyes. Breathe out three times and see yourself holding a glass of clear, pure water. See what happens when a drop of black ink suddenly falls into the water. See and hear the descent of the drop of ink and the rhythm and ripple patterns of the water. Hear what the water is saying to you when it has been hurt or disturbed by the black drop. What are you feeling? Live these feelings deeply by allowing them to fill you. Then wash yourself out by drinking a glass of clear, pure water. Open your eyes, knowing that despair has lifted.

2. Close your eyes. Breathe out three times. Let fall a drop of heavy white ink into the clear, pure water. Look at how far it goes down into the water. See and hear the descent of the drop and the rhythm and ripple patterns of the water. Hear what the water is saying to you when it has been hurt or disturbed by the white drop. What are you feeling? Live these feelings deeply by allowing them to fill you. Then wash yourself out by drinking a glass of clear, pure water. Open your eyes, knowing that despair has lifted.

The Staircase of Life (for depression connected with obsessional [incessantly repetitive] thoughts)

Close your eyes. Breathe out three times. See yourself in a large mansion. See yourself descending the back staircase. Note everything you see and feel. Then see yourself ascending the front staircase. Again note what you see and feel, and when coming to the top, what do you find? Open your eyes.

Blowing Away the Dark Clouds (for a general feeling of blueness)

Close your eyes and see dark clouds above you. As you stand under these clouds, see yourself blowing them away to the left by blowing out three breaths (in imagery, *not* physically). Then look up in the sky to the upper right and watch the sun enter the sky above you. When finished, know that the blues have gone and open your eyes.

Crossing the Bridge (for depression connected with regret)

Close your eyes and breathe out three times. See yourself crossing backward over a bridge. Say good-bye to the ones whom you have loved and who have not done you harm. Ignore the ones who have hurt or harmed you as you cross backward to the other side. When reaching the other side, blow up the bridge between now and the past. Then turn around and see your new shore. Walk on this new shore until you find your new place and feel comforted. You can examine this new abode if you wish. Then open your eyes.

Rebury the Dead (for depression associated with mourning a loved one who has been buried)

Close your eyes. Breathe out three times and see yourself at the cemetery recovering the body of the loved one. See family and friends around you as you rebury the body and then place flowers on the grave. There, recite a short prayer or meditation or good word. Then turn around and see yourself leaving the cemetery, happy, bright, smiling, and reciting a prayer, meditation, or good word. Afterward, breathe out and open your eyes.

The following three exercises for depression associated with loss of energy and motivation use physical activities rather than imagery. I include them because of their ease and effectiveness in remedying this type of depression.

Clean a Space

Physically clean a small area of your home—a sink, mirror, window, floor, desk, etc. Clean it with the intention of cleaning yourself out inside at the same time of your gloom, morbidity or whatever else you choose.

Fingerpainting

Have a drawing pad of unlined white paper. Using fingerpaints of yellow, orange, and red, paint free-form, knowing that your mood is lifting.

Spiral of Energy

In a drawing pad, using a pencil, draw spirals from inside, going out, as in the diagram, any number of times, with the intention of giving yourself energy.

Sailing Out of the Doldrums (for depression connected with being in the doldrums)

You have heard the saying "I'm in the doldrums," meaning that one is feeling blue, sad, or morose. If you experience this malady, then, from an imagery point of view, you

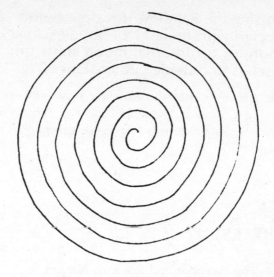

are in luck. This is because the Doldrums do exist. They are located in the Indian Ocean off the coast of Africa, an area of low activity where there is essentially no wind or other kind of turbulence. Now that you know where you are, you can leave.

Close your eyes and breathe out three times, and see yourself sailing in the Doldrums. You are the master of your boat. Know that when you have guided your boat out of the Doldrums, you will feel well. See, feel, and sense how you find your way. Then open your eyes.

Out of Limbo (for depression connected with feeling stuck)

Close your eyes. Breathe out three times and see yourself in limbo. Breathe out once and climb out of limbo. Don't stop until you succeed. Use any means that you find. Remember that this is imagination and *anything* can happen. Then, knowing that you are no longer stuck, open your eyes.

Swallowing the Rainbow (for depression connected with feelings of hopelessness, isolation, or for internal mood shifts not connected to outside circumstances)

Close your eyes. Breathe out three times and see yourself swallowing a rainbow. Sense and feel the uplift this taking in gives you. Stay with this feeling for a minute. Then open your eyes.

DIABETES

Names: **The Acrobat** and **Back to Nature**
Intention: To normalize insulin production in the pancreas.
Frequency: **Acrobat:** Four times a day (before each meal and at bedtime), for three cycles of 21 days of use and 7 days off. In the first week of each cycle do the exercise for 2 to 3 minutes; in the second week, 1 to 2 minutes; in the third week, 30 seconds to 1 minute.
Frequency: **Back to Nature:** Twice a day (in the early morning and at twilight), for 1 to 2 minutes, for as many cycles of 21 days of use and 7 days off as are necessary (sometimes one is enough) to bring the insulin flow into balance.

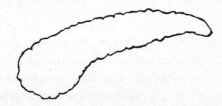

One of the major sugar-regulating chemicals produced in the body is insulin. It is manufactured in the pancreas, a long bridgelike-looking organ located behind the stomach in the upper left region of the abdomen, running from the spleen at the flank to the duodenum (first part of the small intestine) in the middle of the upper abdomen. Diabetes is an illness most often having to do with altered insulin production and glucose (sugar) metabolism. (New research shows that some diabetics are sensitive to processed wheat or saturated fats rather than to refined sugar.) Diabetes is an illness that speaks of *bitterness* in our life. Diabetes calls on us to sweeten our lives, and this can be done by imagining ourselves crossing a bridge from the old bitter life to a new sweeter life. The bridge crossing is specific for diabetes and represents another meaning associated with this illness—that changes must be made if we don't want to get stuck and grow embittered. After doing three cycles of **The Acrobat** or one cycle of **Back to Nature**, check with your doctor to see if your medication needs have changed.

The Acrobat

Close your eyes. Breathe out three times and see yourself crossing over a flowing stream. Become an acrobat, tumbling, jumping, and gyrating your way across, a welcome guest in a new land that awaits you on the other side. Know that your diabetes has subsided when you reach the far shore. Also, give yourself the intention to do something "sweet" for yourself at least once a day.

Back to Nature

Close your eyes. Breathe out three times and see yourself in a meadow. Sit in the middle of this meadow communing with nature and with your higher nature. Know and feel the beauty of both. Breathe out once. Know, feel, and sense the sweetness of life from this contact. Know that your insulin flow is being normalized. Open your eyes when you sense the normal flow.

DIZZINESS

Names: **Tightrope Walking** and **The Acorn**
Intention: To stop dizziness.
Frequency: As needed, for 1 to 2 minutes, every 10 minutes until dizziness is gone.

Dizziness is a common accompaniment to various emotional states, particularly where anxiety or emotional shock is concerned. It can represent our effort to get away from the shock. Most cases of dizziness are short-lived, but some can last for a while. (If dizziness is chronic over three to six months, this may be a sign that some structural disturbance has taken place in the semicircular canals of the inner ear. It is advisable then to consult an ear specialist. You should also see your own doctor for a checkup and reading of your blood pressure.) If you sense yourself becoming dizzy, take a moment to see if you are confused about something, or if you have heard something you didn't want to hear. Try to acknowledge what that might be and try to gather yourself together. Following are two useful imagery exercises for helping to control dizziness.

The exercises are to be done at the first indication of dizziness or when the actual process has started. You can try either one; you don't have to do both.

Tightrope Walking

Close your eyes. Breathe out three times *very slowly*. See and sense yourself as a tightrope walker. Climb the stationary ladder to the platform. On the platform have your pole or bicycle or parasol with you. Before crossing the wire, see yourself reaching the other side. Then begin your crossing, knowing that as you successfully complete this task, your dizziness is disappearing. You may or may not have a net beneath you (your choice). When reaching the other side, to the other platform, put down your pole or bicycle or parasol, and descend the stationary ladder to the ground, knowing that your dizziness has disappeared.

The Acorn

Close your eyes. Breathe out three times *very slowly*. See yourself planting a seed or an acorn in the earth. Breathe out once and sense yourself as this seed or acorn grows as a tree— first as a sprout, then as a sapling, and finally taking root and growing into a tree firmly planted in the earth as your branches reach skyward. Know that you are firmly planted and that your dizziness has disappeared. Then open your eyes.

ECZEMA (see also Skin Disorders)

Name: **Palm Fingers**
Intention: To clear up rash or heal the eczema.
Frequency: Three times a day, for 1 to 3 minutes, for 21 days.

Eczema is a skin disturbance that can cover an enormous area. It is a fierce rash that mirrors the emotional reaction accompanying this process—one of fierce, volcanic anger that cannot find an adequate outlet. Eczema can develop early in life, and it tends to become a chronic ailment, most commonly treated with cortisone, a drug that is not particularly effective in curing the problem. Following is an example of the problem and the treatment I recommended.

"Al," who had been in rage for the last twelve years, was suffering from chronic eczema, which affected his face and many other parts of his body. He had tried many forms of conventional medical treatment without lasting success, and when he came to see me he was using cortisone cream and gaining some relief. However, he agreed to stop using all medication while trying imagery for three weeks.

I prescribed the **Palm Fingers** exercise, which is quite simple.

Palm Fingers

Close your eyes and breathe out three times. See your fingers becoming palm leaves. Put the leaves on your face. Feel the flow of water and milk in them becoming a river of honey that heals the area. Leave a drop of palm oil on the healed area after finishing, seeing your face becoming all clear. Then open your eyes.

Al phoned me a week later; his face had improved considerably, but he was experiencing difficulty with eczema on his body. I instructed him to imagine all ten fingers becoming palm leaves encasing his body so as to swaddle himself in them, and to see his body becoming clear.

Again Al contacted me a week later; his body had cleared up, but he was now experiencing itching. I gave him an imagery exercise in which he was to take off his skin on the banks of a stream, to turn it inside out, and to wash it in the stream, scrubbing the reversed skin with a fine golden brush to cleanse it thoroughly. He was then to turn the skin right-side out and put it back on, knowing that the itching was gone.

One week later, Al reported that the itching had stopped. He also informed me that prior to the imagery work, he would scratch himself at the first sign of an itch because he enjoyed the physical sensation of scratching. The scratching would increase the itch, thus increasing his enjoyment. After the third imagery exercise, he found that he could control this impulse, which was worsening his condition.

During our work together, Al became aware of how the eruption of eczema mirrored his internal eruptions. He was soon able to put his finger (literally and figuratively) on the scene of the eruption. After four weeks of faithfully applying his imaginal "medicine," his skin was perfectly clear, vivid, and free of itching. He had actively undertaken to change and thereby had improved his overall life condition.

In talking with Al three years later, he remarked how helpful and curative the imagery had been. He bemoaned the fact that he didn't have the inner discipline to use the imagery consistently, noting that, when he didn't, the eczema returned.

EDEMA (see Swelling)

EMOTIONAL DISTRESS (including
confusion, disorganization, lack of focus, and terror)

Name: **Meet the Monster**
Intention: To have (name the emotion) disappear.
Frequency: As needed, for 1 to 3 minutes, every 15 to 30 minutes until the emotion is cleared.

Emotional difficulties seem a perpetual accompaniment of living. There are some difficulties that almost everyone encounters: anxiety, worry, anger, guilt, and fear. All emotional difficulties are related to time. That is, we are made uneasy and insecure when we think about the future or the past. It is very difficult to stay centered in the present, as there are endless pressures that push us away from it. As soon as we leave the present, the distressing emotions start, and often they are difficult to control. Following are several simple imagery exercises to help you deal with distress.

As a general rule, distressing emotions are best handled by going toward them, greeting them, entering them, shaking hands with them, going through them, welcoming them, embracing them, or any combination of the above. It is most helpful if you make the attempt to *see* what image is associated with the distressing emotion. Every emotion that can be named has an attendant image that will come to you if you ask for it. Pavlov and his Russian psychologist colleagues proved this point when, in the 1920s, they were working heavily in the area of conditional reflexes and habit patterning. Ivan Pavlov is the best known of these researchers for his salivating dog experiments. Ivan Smolenski demonstrated similar principles in another experiment. Smolenski showed that when a finger flexion is induced by electric shock and conditioned to the sound of a bell for 30 seconds, if the conditional stimulus—the sound of the bell—is replaced by the word "bell," the finger will flex without any other previous preparation.

One patient of mine saw flames connected with the emotion of anger. I asked her to sit in the midst of the flames, letting them flare up around her. At first she was understandably frightened, but eventually she entered into them (probably because she trusted me and, therefore, herself). As she sat in the midst of the flames, she saw their heat taken up by the clouds above her. The clouds became laden with water, burst open, and the rain doused the flames. With this downpour, her anger abruptly ceased. Such experiences are commonplace in my practice.

Another patient was consistently faced with feelings of terror. I asked her to see the terror, which she envisioned as a ghost with horrifying dark eyes and surrounded by flames. She went toward this figure rather than retreating. She then went through the figure and found herself on the other side in a beautiful green meadow. The sun was shining brightly, the sky was light blue, the trees quite green. She felt a sense of peace, and the feeling of terror evaporated. She repeated this experience each time she felt terrified. Within two weeks, being "terrified" became a thing of the past for her.

I offer this technique as a general way to handle unsettling emotions. The first step is not to give in to the emotion. Don't be intimidated or scared by it. The emotion wants you to do its bidding. It's like a little mental child clamoring for attention and feeding. What I am suggesting as an approach amounts to ignoring it and starving it in the long run.

Meet the Monster

Close your eyes and breathe out once. In whatever way is appropriate, go to your emotion and see the image associated with it. Know that what happens in this confrontation will relieve you. Open your eyes when finished.

EMOTIONAL WOUNDS

Name: **Personal Odyssey**
Intention: To heal emotional wounds.
Frequency: Once, for 5 to 10 minutes. If needed, use once a
   month.

Emotional wounds don't need a lengthy description. We have all suffered them at one time or another. We all know that they can take a long time to heal and that they can leave scars, like physical wounds. Fortunately, the passage of time is a great healer for these wounds. The following imagery exercise can facilitate this healing process.

Personal Odyssey

Close your eyes. Breathe out once. Find yourself at the base of a cliff at a beach. Know how you've gotten to the base of the cliff. Then look at the white cliff and, with a sharp stone, engrave all the negative feelings that have been plaguing you and bothering you. Engrave those traits deeply into the stone. Then lay out a white sail on the beach. Take a hammer and large rocks. Break up the traits by throwing rocks at the cliff where you have engraved them. Then take the hammer and finish the job. See the stone breaking up and falling from the cliff. Gather the pieces in the white sail and tie it up by putting together the four corners to make a bag. Gather together wood taken from shipwrecks at the bottom of the sea, and make a boat. Start the boat from the shore where you are located geographically in your part of the country. Go through waterways, meeting the people of different countries and relating to them by adapting a different response from the habitual trait(s) in the bag. Eventually, turn your boat into the Pacific Ocean and go to the deepest part, and there drop the bag, seeing it disappear from view underwater. Come back feeling lighter, and sail the boat in the opposite direction through the Pacific, back through the waterways, stopping along the way to learn about the people and understand them, having been paci-fied in the Pacific. Return to the shore from which you started. Then look at the fresh cliff, having a sharp tip of metal pressing in your hand to remind you not to touch this freshness. Then jump to the top of the cliff with your new lightness and there, in a meadow, let yourself be quiet and relax. Afterward, open your eyes.

ENDING A RELATIONSHIP

Name: **The Sands of Time**
Intention: To end the relationship (to a specified person).
Frequency: Twice a day (early morning and twilight) for up
to 3 minutes, for 7 days.

Name: **Parting and Departing**
Intention: To end the influence of a person in your life; to
end the relationship.
Frequency: Each morning, for 3 to 5 minutes, for 7 days.

One of the situations I often encounter in my practice is the
suffering experienced in not being able to end a relationship. This is a situation in which a severing of ties is
desired, but, for any of a number of reasons, the person can't
make the necessary break. Here are two tried and true ways
to bring this about for yourself. The second might be
considered more severe than the first. Use the one that suits
you.

The Sands of Time

Close your eyes. Breathe out three times and see yourself
walking along a beach holding hands with the one with
whom you are ending. The two of you are dancing, skip-
ping, and cavorting along the beach. Then you drop hands,
say good-bye, and *retrace* your steps *backward,* cleaning out
thoroughly everything that you see before you. See and
sense your effort. Finally, you reach the shoreline. The
waves wash up on the beach, clearing away all the residue of
the relationship that remains. You then swim out to the
horizon, using a regular crawl stroke, seeing your arms and
legs becoming very long and your torso elongating. Breathe
in the pure air from the horizon. Meet the horizon and
come back to shore using a backstroke, your arms stretched
out far behind your head, your legs stretched out far in

front of you, kicking. Your torso, too, is elongated. Keep breathing the pure air from the horizon. When reaching the shore, come out and let the sun dry you. Then, put on a clean robe or gown that you find there, and return to your home. Then open your eyes.

Parting and Departing

Close your eyes. Breathe out three times and see yourself on a beach. The one with whom you wish to end is lying there. You have with you golden ropes with lead weights at the ends. With these you truss up your "friend". There is a large rowboat nearby. You shove the boat off and put your "friend" in it; get in and row out to the Marianas Trench off the Philippines, one of the deepest spots in the world. Stand up in the boat, lift your "friend's" trussed-up body, and toss it overboard, knowing that you are *ridding yourself of the influence* of that person. Watch the body disappear as it sinks, forming a small whirlpool. Know that it is going to the bottom, never to surface again. After it has gone out of sight, sit down in the boat and row back to shore with a new feeling and attitude about yourself. When you reach the shore, stow the oars and beach the boat, and return to your home alone. Then open your eyes.

EPSTEIN-BARR VIRUS (chronic fatigue syndrome)

Name: **The Polo Pony**
Intention: To eliminate the virus.
Frequency: Three times a day, for 3 minutes, for nine cycles of 21 days of use and 7 days off. By the seventh cycle, 1 minute for this exercise is sufficient. Intervening medical tests are helpful if you desire them, but they are not

mandatory (some people do not want to be mentally tied to the results of white-cell-count testing).

The occurrence of this viral infection has caused alarm because certain research findings suggest that it could be a forerunner of certain forms of cancer and of AIDS. Some people consider the Epstein-Barr virus to be a version of the herpes genitalia virus. People with Epstein-Barr feel excessive fatigue and become physically debilitated. Such symptoms really indicate a general rundown condition that provides a perfect medium for the virus to attack. My view is that organisms such as viruses, bacteria, or any other microbes don't cause illness. They are the result of altered conditions within us that provide the necessary environment for these organisms to grow. In those individuals I've seen who were diagnosed as having Epstein-Barr virus, it has been quite clear that their life situations, at the time of occurrence, had been somewhat overwhelming. In one instance, a young man gave so much of himself in a relationship that he left himself thoroughly depleted of energy, becoming vulnerable to infection through a weakening of his immune system. In another situation, a young woman tested her endurance to the limit by driving herself at her job in order to get promoted and climb the corporate ladder. These two people taught me much about what I might offer as practical therapeutic steps to help combat this condition.

The illustration here was done by one of my patients who sought to depict his Epstein-Barr virus. He sketched the invader(s) being attacked by an army of "good guys" in the form of white blood cells that looked like voracious piranña fish. Some of the cells had the label BHT, a medical product he was taking to help combat the virus. Immediately after completing the drawing, the man experienced a sense of physical and emotional well-being. As he continued looking at this picture over the following weeks, he experienced the same sensation of well-being. I encouraged him to keep the picture where he could see it often, to serve as a

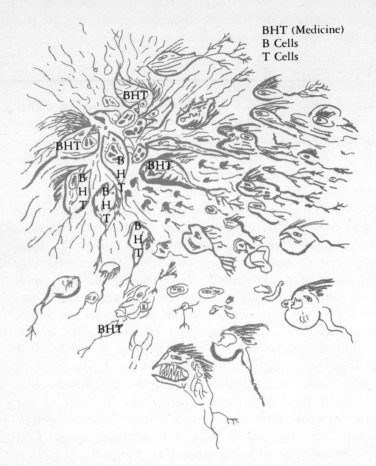

BHT (Medicine)
B Cells
T Cells

reminder of his intention to destroy the invaders by his "protecting army." In essence, he is re-membering his wholeness. This process of using an external reminder to stimulate an internal response was a characteristic treatment in Western medicine for a thousand or more years. Then it was abandoned for the past three centuries, but now it is finding its way back into the mainstream through the field of biofeedback.

Drawing is the external expression of what has been going on inside. Once it is depicted on the outside, it can be used to stimulate the inner process in a different way, by imparting a new message to the inner self. This reciprocal relationship forms a special kind of feedback system, which in turn helps to promote the healing function of imagery, which reminds patients of their intention to heal themselves.

Regardless of whether you suffer from trouble that expresses itself physically or emotionally or both, and regardless of whether you can draw well (your skill at drawing is absolutely irrelevant), *see* what your malady looks like and draw it. No matter how ridiculous what you see turns out, draw it! Afterward, on that same paper, destroy, imprison, encase, or otherwise contain your malady to the best of your ability, and then use it with the *intention* of fighting and healing your trouble. Getting a sense of the effectiveness of this method will alert you to the strength and power of imagination.

To reiterate, the system works to:

1. Make outside what's inside
2. Reshape what's been made outside
3. Use the outside to remind the inside of its purpose

The inner action gives us a sense of well-being that prompts us to use the outside form again to give instructions to the inside. This instruction takes the form of an image (picture) rather than words.

One young woman with Epstein-Barr virus devised a number of powerful imagery exercises, which I have incorporated along with imagery designed to help stimulate the immune function. I offer here one exercise that she developed, which has proved extremely helpful for any virus, such as Epstein-Barr, that weakens the immune system.

The Polo Pony

Close your eyes, breathe out three times, and go into your body. See yourself playing a flute while riding a polo pony and carrying a polo mallet in your saddle. Lure the viruses out of the tissues by playing your choice of music, then kill the viruses with your mallet. Then open your eyes.

FARSIGHTEDNESS and NEARSIGHTEDNESS

Name: **Boat in the Harbor**
Intention: To correct visual defects.
Frequency: In the morning for 3 to 6 minutes. If you can,
    try to do the exercise a second time each day, at twilight.

Farsightedness has to do with not seeing details clearly—
seeing the forest and not the trees. Nearsightedness has to
do with seeing details but not having a grasp of the larger
picture—seeing the trees but not the forest. Astigmatism
denotes some confusion about someone or something—not
seeing clearly; it is evident in both near- and farsightedness.
Following is the imagery for nearsightedness. For farsightedness, simply reverse the direction. As the eyesight begins
to improve, so does the astigmatism.

Boat in the Harbor

Close your eyes. Breathe out three times and see yourself
standing in a harbor. In the distance is a steamship. See the
ship begin to move to your left. It sails in a circle from your
left all the way around your head to the right and comes
back to the center. Do not physically move your head while
watching the ship, but imaginally turn and swivel your eyes
as far as you can to follow the boat. Then see the boat come
into the harbor toward you, turn around, and sail out to the
horizon. Have the boat now turn to the right and sail
around you in a complete circle to the left, coming back to
the center of the horizon. (Again, your *imaginal* eyes follow
its movement.) The boat then sails into the harbor toward
you and turns around to go back out to the horizon. From
the stacks of the ship, see a flock of birds fly off toward you
and follow them with your imaginal eyes, again keeping
your head still, till they fly just overhead and behind your

head. They turn around and fly back toward the ship and beyond the ship into the distance, disappearing from sight. Afterward, breathe out and open your eyes.

For farsightedness, the ship should start in the harbor and sail out to the horizon, then circle both left and right around your head, ending up back in the harbor. The birds should fly from the stacks directly out to the horizon and then return toward you and behind you, returning then to the stacks before you breathe out and open your eyes.

FEAR

Name: **23rd Psalm** and **Reversing Gravity**
Intention: To stop fear.
Frequency: As needed, for 1 to 2 minutes, every 15 to 30 minutes until fear subsides.

Name: **The King**
Intention: To stop fear.
Frequency: As needed, up to 1 minute, every 15 to 30 minutes until fear subsides.

Name: **The Eight-Cornered Room**
Intention: To stop fear.
Frequency: Four times a day (morning, noon, twilight, and bedtime), for 2 to 3 minutes, for 7 days.

Name: **Keep the Faith** and **Fear Fear!**
Intention: To stop fear.
Frequency: As needed, for 30 seconds, every 15 to 30 minutes until fear subsides.

The major antagonist to faith or trust is fear. Fear always relates to something or someone external to ourselves, in contrast to anxiety (see p. 59), which is generated from within. The human basic fear is that of the dark. The two key offshoots of this fundamental fear relate to apprehension about the unknown and about death (the latter usually appears between the ages of 6 and 8). The exaggeration of fear is called *phobia*.

My clinical experience has shown me that fear is largely a consequence of some thought or action that we believe is not morally appropriate or correct. In truth, we create fear ourselves by our beliefs. Acknowledge where you may be contributing to your own fear, because to know this is to know that what you create you may "de-create." You made it, so you can also unmake it. Don't respond by thinking that I am making you feel guilty for putting such an onus or burden on you. Just know that in becoming your own authority you have to assume authorship. You have to know how you create your own enslavement if you are going to create your own freedom. Doing this actually brings relief.

I contrasted fear to faith above because it is not common to find people of trust beset by fear. King David, in the 23rd Psalm, beautifully expressed the antidote to fear when he said, "Yea, though I walk through the valley of the shadow of death, I shall fear no evil, for thou art with me; thy rod and thy staff they comfort me . . . my cup runneth over."

Here are some possibilities for gaining mastery over fear reactions. Some of the exercises are quite brief. An axiom of successful imaging is that less is more. This is because imagery works by giving a jolt to our mental and physical systems to stimulate their innate healing functions. Use any or all of them anytime you require it.

23rd Psalm

Close your eyes. Breathe out three times. See yourself carrying your rod and staff. Use your staff to help you walk a straight road, and use your rod to knock away any fearful image that intrudes on your path. Then see your cup overflowing. Open your eyes, knowing that fear has gone.

Reversing Gravity

Close your eyes. Breathe out once. You are about to be engulfed by an unknown force. See it! Then reverse gravitation and fly above and away from it. As you do, your fear leaves. Then open your eyes.

The King

Each time you feel afraid, close your eyes and see the face of a king, or some courageous person you know. Then become one with that person for an instant. Open your eyes, knowing that fear has disappeared.

The Eight-Cornered Room

Close your eyes. Breathe out three times. Clean the eight corners of a room (four below, four above) thoroughly. Don't stop until all the dirt is cleaned. Then open your eyes, knowing that fear has gone.

Keep the Faith

Close your eyes. Breathe out once. Change fear to faith. See and keep this image for yourself. Open your eyes.

Fear Fear!

Close your eyes. Breathe out once. Fear fear! Now go from awful to awe! Open your eyes.

FEELING ILL

Name: **The Bronze Serpent**
Intention: To overcome feeling ill.
Frequency: Once a day, for 1 to 2 minutes, for 7 days.

I like to use "feeling ill" instead of *hypochondria*, because that word carries the implication that the sufferer is *not really* experiencing something genuinely physical. We should never discount a physical complaint even if we can't find physical evidence of it. Feeling ill is a genuine way of responding in the world, and we must be tolerant, accepting, and unbiased to acknowledge it. Following is an imagery exercise designed to help you accept the experience and to feel better.

The Bronze Serpent

Close your eyes. Breathe out three times. See the bronze serpent atop the pole held by Moses. Look into its eyes and know the healing that is taking place in you. Then open your eyes.

FRIGIDITY

Name: **The Blue Cocoon**
Intention: To become sexually responsive.
Frequency: Once a day for 3 minutes, for 8 days.

Frigidity is the female counterpart of impotence. It is characterized by a woman's inability to experience vaginal sensation during intercourse or to achieve a climax. Volumes have been written about the emotional implications of frigidity. Indeed, it can be valuable to investigate the emotional/

social issues, as well as the physical ones, that are at work in this problem. However, for the immediate problem of frigidity, **The Blue Cocoon** should prove helpful.

The Blue Cocoon

Close your eyes. Breathe out three times. See yourself going into a cave where you encounter a monster. See yourself fighting and killing the monster. Then skin it. Return to the entrance of the cave, and exit taking the skin of the monster with you. Once outside, meet your man, go to a meadow and sit with him under a tree. The blue-golden light of the cloudless blue sky and bright golden sun is taken in by both of you. Then see the two of you in a cocoon of blue light, and see and feel what happens. See the blue light permeating all your own blood cells as well as the sperm of your partner. Then open your eyes.

CHRONIC GASTROINTESTINAL DISTURBANCES

Name: **Inside-Outside**
Intention: To heal the (name of disturbance).
Frequency: Twice a day, early morning and at bedtime, for
   3 to 5 minutes, for six cycles of 21 days of use and 7 days
   off. If you need feedback, check with your physician after
   the third cycle to get an indication of your progress. Do
   not discontinue your medications before checking with
   your doctor.

Name: **The Mermaid**
Intention: To heal the (name of disturbance).
Frequency: Three times a day, early morning, twilight, and
   at bedtime, for up to 3 minutes, for three cycles of 21
   days of use and 7 days off.

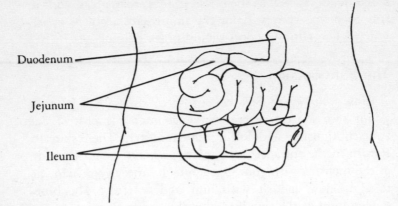

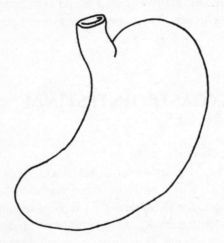

Intestinal disturbances include upsets that affect the stomach, any of the three parts of the small intestine (duodenum, jejunum, ileum), and the colon, rectum, or anus (as shown in the diagram). Many of these difficulties are connected with poor eating habits and/or overdrinking and are relatively minor, while others can be of a more serious nature—such as peptic ulcer, which affects either the stomach or the duodenum.

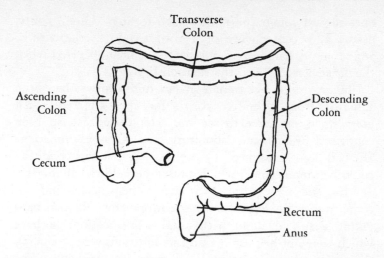

Each part of the intestine reflects an emotional process and has a critical meaning in our lives. The esophagus has the meaning of being able to "swallow" something, literally or figuratively. The stomach deals with being able to "stomach" something or not. The duodenum and jejunum have to do with control, usually concerns about controlling others. The ileum reflects feelings of inferiority or insecurity about ourselves or about the positions we hold in life. The large intestine (including the rectum and anus) often concerns issues of hatred, deep resentment, or deeply held bitterness, as well as prolonged holding on to lost love relationships, which is analogous to prolonged mourning.

Colitis is a commonly diagnosed illness affecting the large bowel. This chronic inflammation of the lower bowel, for which medical treatments, including the commonly used cortisone prescription, are not terribly effective, comes in many forms. Spastic, ulcerative, and mucous are some of the labels given to it, depending on the severity and involvement of the large bowel. Whatever the type, colitis has much to do with issues regarding holding on and not letting go, and with feelings of hatred or deep resentment. Here it is important for you to be able to forgive the one or ones toward whom you harbor such feelings. Often, colitis occurs as a consequence of a thwarted love relationship, where one is hanging on to the resentment incurred when the other person ended the relationship.

"Linda," a young woman in her midtwenties, had been suffering from ulcerative colitis for approximately seven years when she came to see me. Her diagnosis had been confirmed by physical, laboratory, and X-ray examination. She had been "informed" by a physician that this condition could be precancerous, which caused her additional anxiety. She had tried "everything" in order to help herself and had come to me on referral from her chiropractor. She had been taking a steroid along with another medication, both of which were not helping her and in addition were producing their own adverse reactions. We went immediately to the point of trouble and began by using the two exercises described below, **Inside-Outside** and **The Mermaid**. Over a span of three months, diligently dedicating herself to using imagery, Linda found a number of shifts taking place in her life: she stopped using her medication while she was under my care, and her disease process ceased, proved by X-ray examination; she became more assertive in her life in general, overcoming anxiety about performing in front of audiences; and she established a satisfying and secure relationship with a young man with whom she began to live. Holding on to lost love relationships and acknowledging feelings of hatred emerged during the course of our work together; once she was able to let go, she was healed.

In the main, imagery has been successful with gastrointestinal conditions and their associated emotional turbulence. Following are two excellent imagery exercises that can be used for any of these problems.

Inside-Outside

Close your eyes. Breathe out three times and see yourself by a fast-flowing, crystal-clear mountain stream. Kneel down by this stream, reach into your abdomen, and pull out the part of the intestinal tract that is impaired. Turn it inside out and wash it thoroughly in the stream, using a fine-bristled golden brush to clear out all the waste and debris, seeing all the injured material being washed away downstream by the cool, rushing water. Afterward, take the intestinal part out of the water and place it on the fertile earth by the bank, letting it dry in the sun, filling the area with light. When dry, take a fine golden needle, thread it with find golden thread, and repair any damage by weaving the walls of the injured tract, sensing the edges of the wall coming together so that you see all traces of injury disappearing. See the newly repaired segment looking normal and healthy. Then gently massage the exposed part with downward strokes, sensing the blood flowing evenly through it, and tell it that you love it. Then turn it right side out and place it back in your abdomen. Then take in some nutritious food. Digest it as a snake does, experiencing it passing through your digestive tube as it is in the process of being perfectly digested. At the end, see this fully digested material eliminated as a perfectly formed fecal mass, knowing that your intestinal tract is performing perfectly. Then open your eyes.

The Mermaid

Close your eyes. Breathe out three times. See a mermaid with golden hair and a silvery blue body and tail. See and sense her traveling through your intestinal tract in a rhythmical manner. Have her touch the area of the tract where you have the disturbance, and see the area healing completely. Have her complete the journey through the tract, making sure everything else is in order. When she has completed her journey, breathe out and open your eyes.

GLAUCOMA

Name: **The Canal of Schlemm**
Intention: To bring your intraocular pressure to normal.
Frequency: Three times a day, for 1 to 3 minutes, for
  21 days. Then use the exercise once a day until you feel
  you have the situation well in hand.

Glaucoma is an eye malady in which there is insufficient
drainage of fluid called the aqueous humor in the area
surrounding the lens, an area called the posterior and anterior
chamber. When this drainage doesn't occur, there is a
buildup of pressure that can lead to serious eye impairment
and eventually to loss of vision and blindness. It is beneficial to study the diagram of the eye to familiarize yourself
with the drainage channels, for they are important in this
exercise. Additionally, it is necessary to know that the pupil
of the eye acts similarly to the diaphragm, which helps us
breathe. The pupil, however, opens and closes instead of
contracting and expanding, as the diaphragm does. As with
most eye problems we encounter, the emotional/ social issue
of what it is we don't want to see, or what we have been
blind to, has to be taken into account. Pursuing some of the
emotional and social issues connected with this eye ailment
can also be of great value as preventive work, since it helps
you prepare to look your trouble in the eye.

"Bernard" had been suffering from glaucoma for nearly
eight years when he first visited me. His intraocular pressure was being monitored on a regular basis by his ophthalmologist, who prescribed three medications taken together
to keep the pressure within normal limits. The ophthalmologist agreed to continue as Bernard's primary physician and
monitor his intraocular pressure and progress during the
three-week program of imagery I developed for him. During the course of our work together, I asked Bernard to
discontinue the medications he was taking for his glaucoma.

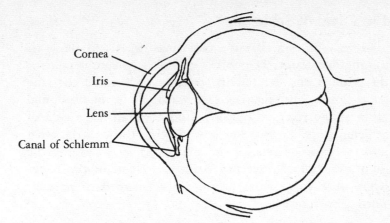

Cornea

Iris

Lens

Canal of Schlemm

Aqueous humor probably is filtered out of the blood in the capillaries of the ciliary body and may also be actively secreted by these vessels. Once it is produced, aqueous humor moves into the posterior chamber, and from there moves between the lens and iris, through the pupil, and into the anterior chamber. From the anterior chamber, it normally moves into a narrow channel that passes like a ring through the anterior part of the schlera, the Canal of Schlemm. This canal acts as a venous sinus, draining the humor into numerous small veins.

The doctor, although somewhat uncomfortable about this, agreed to see if imagery alone would be effective. As a reinforcement for his imaging, Bernard looked at a picture of the eye area that he was going to be visualizing.

Bernard used **The Canal of Schlemm** for 3 weeks, 3 times a day, for 1 to 3 minutes. At the end of that time, his ophthalmologist checked his pressure and found it had remained normal without medication. I spoke to Bernard five years later, when he told me he still used the imagery and one of the three medications to maintain his normal intraocular pressure. He also said that he has used imagery successfully, after being introduced to this possibility in our work, to help him successfully in emotionally critical situations he has since encountered.

The Canal of Schlemm

Close your eyes. Breathe out three times and sense air coming in through the pupil of your eye. As you breathe in, the pupil opens, lets air in, and as you breathe out, the pupil closes. Sense the air creating a ripple in the fluid, and pushing the river of aqueous fluid through the Canal of Schlemm. Feel the wave of fluid flowing through the canal into the adjacent venous sinus (opening), and carrying the fluid away into the venous drainage system of the body. Know that your ocular pressure has returned to normal. Then open your eyes.

GRIEF

Name: **Change of Heart**
Intention: To remove grief.
Frequency: Every 1 to 2 hours while awake, for 1 to 2
    minutes, for 7 days, or less if grieving stops before then.

Grief is a normal, natural, and often necessary response to loss/separation. The shock of such severing brings forth this eruptive, organismic, overwhelming emotional outburst. Such a response is our way of trying to heal from the shock, and we need not shy away from it. Grief reactions are usually followed by a longer period of mourning, where the reactions are less acute. Following is an imagery exercise to help you go through that process.

Change of Heart

Close your eyes. Breathe out three times. See your heart. Zip open your chest and take out your heart. Clean it gently and afterwards, throw it into the cosmos. Retrieve it from the comos and see that it's a crystal heart. Invite all the people you love to enter it, smiling and bright; be aware that you can see them there always. Put your crystal heart back into place, zip up your chest, then open your eyes, knowing that your grief is relieved.

GUILT

Name: **The Red Ribbon** and **Speaking Your Mind**
Intention: To eliminate guilt feelings.
Frequency: Once a day, for 3 to 5 minutes (for **Speaking Your Mind,** up to 3 minutes only), for 7 days. If you feel you need to go on, continue for another 14 days.

Much is made of guilt feelings, which are often associated with our sense of conscience. Actually, conscience is present in some, though not all, of us to prevent us from carrying out destructive acts against ourselves or others. Technically speaking what we feel after committing an act that goes against our conscience is remorse, although we commonly call that guilt. Conscience prevents us from committing such acts beforehand. Remorse as "guilt feelings" is a response after the fact. Call this response what you will, these feelings stifle personal growth, for they are a way of ducking responsibility for behavior that you've undertaken, or for behavior that you have not undertaken. In other words, we not only feel guilty for what we have done, but for what we haven't done. In either case, don't keep yourself rooted to the past. Take responsibility for your action of doing or not doing. Know that there are consequences for your actions that you have to bear, forgive yourself, ask the one you have hurt or offended for forgiveness. Make compensation, if you can, and go on living in the present, trying to act as ethically as you can.

The following exercises have been powerful allies in the fight that many of my patients have undergone in order to escape the paralyzing grip of guilt feelings. Find which of the exercises suits you and stick with it. It is amazing what you'll find out about yourself through exploring guilt in this way.

The Red Ribbon

Close your eyes. Breathe out three times. See a red ribbon in front of you. Write on this ribbon the traits you want to be rid of, including guilt. List these traits in the order of importance they hold for you. Put the ribbon around your neck. Breathe out once and go from the city into the desert—one that you have seen or read about. Find there a waterfall that has a large rock nearby. In front of the rock dig a hole. Take all the traits from the ribbon and expel them one by one by breathing out while naming each trait (not out loud but *there* in the desert). Afterward, place the ribbon on the rock and burn it. Place the ashes in the hole; fill in the hole and place the rock on top. Breathe out once and go to the waterfall. Climb from the bottom to the top, straight up the cascading water itself. See, feel, and sense the force of the water rushing over you, cleansing you, and washing away any residual guilt. After reaching the top, hold your hands, palms up, toward the sun, taking some of it in your hands and then placing them anywhere you wish on or in your body to give you health and well-being. Breathe out once and come out of the waterfall. Let the sun dry you. Put on a clean robe or gown and return to your chair knowing your guilt has gone. Then open your eyes.

Speaking Your Mind

Close your eyes. Breathe out three times. Imagine yourself speaking to the person who is in conflict with you about the very thing for which you are feeling guilty. Express yourself directly, saying whatever it is you feel guilty about.

Then change places with the other person. Become this other person and talk to yourself as if you were this other person. Breathe out once. Then return to being yourself and express to the other person the resentment that lies behind the guilt. Breathe out once. Now change places and respond to what you have felt. Breathe out once. Become yourself again and express the demands that lie behind this resentment. Don't disguise your demands as questions or accusations. Breathe out once. Be the other person and respond to the demands you have just made. Note how you feel physically when you change places. As the other person, what do you say? Then open your eyes.

HEADACHES

Name: **The Silver Band**
Intention: To eliminate temporal headaches.
Frequency: Every 5 to 10 minutes, for 1 to 2 minutes, until the headache disappears.

Name: **Open Eyes**
Intention: To eliminate migraine headaches.
Frequency: As needed when headache occurs, for 2 to 3 minutes.

Name: **Lake of the Brain**
Intention: To eliminate tension headaches.
Frequency: As needed, every 5 to 10 minutes, for up to 3 minutes.

These are the three of the most commonly experienced of the wide variety of headaches that exist. The diagram shows the three main sites for the headaches I'm describing.

Headaches are characteristically related to one's emotional state. Temporal headaches involve rage; migraine headaches involve anger; tension headaches involve worry. Temporal

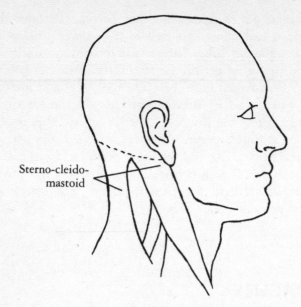

Sterno-cleido-
mastoid

headache is experienced as that "pounding in my head"
where there is great pressure felt at both sides of the head in
the region of the temporal bones. It can arise when you do
not allow yourself to say what you feel. Migraine headache
is usually felt as one-sided, the pain covering the entire
surface of that side of the skull; its onset is often signaled by
the sensation of smelling something unpleasant (unrelated
to what is in the environment) or seeing a halo of colored
lights (also unrelated to environmental presence), and most
commonly reflects anger. Tension headache is muscular in
origin and mirrors the tension you feel in your life. It is
experienced at the base of the skull and in the large muscles
of the neck fitted into the base of the skull.

The Silver Band (for temporal headaches)

Close your eyes. Breathe out three times and imagine a
silver band stretched tightly across your skull from temporal

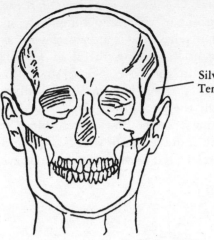

Silver band over
Temporal Bones

bone to temporal bone and flaring out slightly at the ends as it lies on the bones.

See and sense the band tightening around your skull, with the ends pressing against the temporal bones and then quickly releasing; the band and ends squeeze once again and then release quickly; and again a third time. Then open your eyes, knowing that the pain has gone.

Open Eyes (for migraine headaches)

With your eyes open, look up and out to the side of the headache for 2 to 3 minutes steadily. Then return to your normal gaze.

Lake of the Brain (for tension headaches)

Close your eyes and breathe out three times. Look down at the top of your head. Lift off the top of your skull as if you were removing the top of the shell of a soft-boiled egg. Look inside. See the fluid of your brain and the moving nerve fibers that look like water plants underneath. See the fluid draining out of your head completely and sense and feel the tension relieved at the base of your skull and the back of your neck, sensing the fluid moving down the spinal column to the base. See fresh fluid moving up the spinal column, through the neck, and filling your skull, seeing through the clean, clear liquid to the nerve fibers below. Feel and sense the flow of fresh blood through your neck and down into the rest of your body. Put on the top of your skull, breathe out once, and open your eyes.

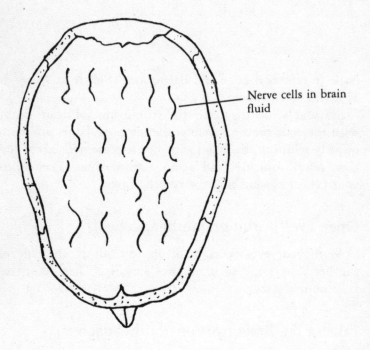

Nerve cells in brain fluid

HEMORRHOIDS (piles)

Name: **The Puckered Purse**
Intention: To eliminate hemorrhoids.
Frequency: Every hour, for 1 to 2 minutes, for up to 21 days or until the hemorrhoids disappear.

Hemorrhoids are outcroppings or outpocketings of blood vessels in the anus. They are either external or internal. The former lie under the skin outside the anal opening; the latter lie under the surface of the lining at the anal canal. In either case, my experience has been that when hemorrhoids are present, the sufferers are responding to unexpressed anger and resentment, particularly the latter. They are holding on and in too much. This imagery exercise should be helpful.

The Puckered Purse

Close your eyes. Breathe out three times. See and sense your hemorrhoid(s) becoming puckered like an old purse, then shriveling and finally disappearing, the anus walls becoming pink and smooth. Then open your eyes.

HERPES GENITALIA

Name: **Snake Hunting** and **The Serpent of Illness**
Intention: To heal yourself of herpes.
Frequency: Twice a day for **Snake Hunting**, three times a day for **The Serpent of Illness**, for 21 days; for 2 to 3 minutes the first week, 1 to 2 minutes the second week, and 30 seconds to 1 minute the third week. After the cycle of 21 days of use followed by 7 days off, get reexamined by your doctor. Enjoy the clean bill of health.

If you have not improved, continue the process (with the same exercise) for another two cycles of 21 days on and 7 days off. Get another checkup after completing the third cycle.

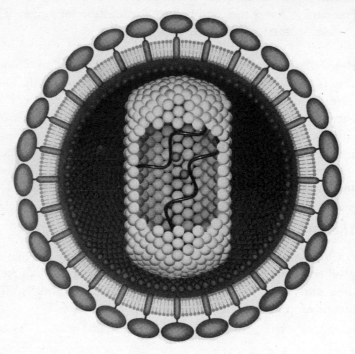

credit George V. Kelvin

Herpes genitalia is a venereal disease that is often chronic in both sexes. In some women it comes and goes with the menstrual cycle, but in others it remains chronic throughout the month. *Herpes* means "snake," and it is this meaning that gives a key to finding the imagery to help stem its course.

The herpes virus is a cousin of the AIDS virus, which was pictured on the cover of the January 1987 *Scientific American*. Looking at this diagram, I was struck at seeing two serpents in the center of the virus surrounded by what appears to be an impregnable fortress of symmetrically placed cells. I include this picture because it may encourage you to emulate Saint Patrick, and imaginally drive the snakes out of your body.

Following are two exercises that I have used. The first, **Snake Hunting,** is also useful for AIDS.

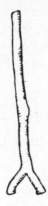

Snake Hunting

Close your eyes. Breathe out three times. You are wearing your special snake-hunting outfit. You have with you your golden snake-catching stick with two prongs at the end, as in the diagram above. Enter the maze of illness, carrying with you a ball of golden thread, which you unravel to help you find your way back. Breathe out once and find your way to the center of the maze, trailing the thread behind you. At the center, catch the snake(s) using your snake-catching stick. Put it (them) in your special golden burlap bag and secure the top. Breathe out once and find your way back to the beginning of the maze. After emerging, take the bag to an altar in an open field, or to a temple (whichever you prefer). Burn the bag and its contents as an offering to the universe. Know that the universe gladly accepts the offering. Take the ashes and scatter them to the winds behind you. Then open your eyes.

The Serpent of Illness

Close your eyes. Breathe out three times and see the serpent of your illness snaking toward you, coming to curse you. Breathe out once and *throw* a curse back at this serpent that has come to curse you. Breathe out once and, like Saint Patrick, follow the movements of the serpent without distraction, and know that in so doing you are cleaning out the curse that has been put in you as you sense and feel that you are putting yourself in order. Then open your eyes.

HYPERTENSION (high blood pressure)

Name: **Ice Cubes** and **The Healing Sun**
Intention: To bring your blood pressure to normal.
Frequency: Three times a day, and whenever you sense your pressure is elevated, for 3 to 5 minutes.

Name: **Becoming Part of Nature**
Intention: To bring your blood pressure to normal, or to maintain stabilized blood pressure.
Frequency: Three times a day, and whenever you sense your pressure is elevated, for 3 minutes.

High blood pressure is usually associated with anxiety, anger, and ambition. As we push ourselves to satisfy our desires, we find ourselves "burning up." In hypertension, our blood and anger are boiling over and have to be cooled down. Try to look at the combination of factors that can play a role in high blood pressure. Emotional and dietary problems are of major concern, as well as your overall life situation. You might recognize that your diet is directly connected to your emotional life. And salt, which is directly implicated in blood pressure elevation, can be an addictive agent.

In 1986, the National Institutes of Health announced that the first treatment it would recommend for high blood pressure is meditation—that is, they recommend using your mind before using drugs to control your blood pressure.

Many people with high blood pressure can often internally sense when their pressure is high. Any one of these exercises can be used when you know that your pressure is elevated. Test all to find the one that works best for you.

Ice Cubes

Close your eyes, breathe out three times, and imagine yourself going to your refrigerator and taking out three or four ice cubes. Wash your head, skull, face, and neck with the ice, and sense and feel the coolness coursing through every pore and entering into your bloodstream in the brain. See this ice-blue coolness circulating down from the brain through the neck, down into your trunk, into and through your upper and lower extremities, and out to the tips of your fingers and toes. Know that when you see and sense this ice-blue coolness reaching to your fingertips and toes, your blood pressure has returned to normal. Then open your eyes.

Do this exercise slowly, making sure that you *sense* the flow of blueness as well as see it at each level.

The Healing Sun

Close your eyes. Breathe out three times and see, sense, and feel sunlight entering you from above. The sun's rays enter into your upper arms and upper thighs. See, sense, and feel these rays moving down slowly through every segment of your upper arms and upper thighs, sensing the warmth of the rays as you do so. Then see the rays go through your elbows and knees and on into the upper segments of your forearms and calves. Proceed down them very slowly, seeing, sensing, and feeling the sun's rays, knowing that as you do so, your pressure is returning to normal. This process is continued through your wrists and ankles and into your hands and feet, ending with sensing, seeing, and feeling the warmth at your fingertips and toes. When you sense warmth in all of your fingers and toes, open your eyes.

Becoming Part of Nature

Close your eyes, breathe out three times, and see yourself entering any place in nature that is restful for you. Wherever you find yourself, see and sense yourself becoming part of the environment and part of the rhythm of the environment. If you are at the seashore, touch the sand and let it sift through your fingers. See the cloudless blue sky and bright golden sun, which you feel beating down on you and warming you. Smell the fresh ocean air, and listen to the waves lapping up onto the shore. Find yourself coming into harmony with the movement of the waves, and as you do so, know that your blood pressure is returning to normal. Then open your eyes.

IMMUNE SUPPRESSION

Name: **The Artist of Life**

Intention: To help yourself heal by increasing positive immune function.

Frequency: Six times a day, or every 2 hours (if you can't manage this schedule, then do it five times a day or every 3 hours), for 3 minutes, for any number of cycles of 21 days on and 7 days off, until the immune function becomes stabilized in terms of symptom removal and/or white blood cell counts.

The immune system has become prominent in our consciousness recently because of the publicity given to AIDS and cancer. Imagery used to stimulate the immune system almost invariably raises the immune level in any disorder in which it is lowered. Those patients whom I've treated for AIDS or ARC (AIDS-related complex) consistently show elevations of their white blood cell counts after imagery. While the immune system certainly helps to protect us from the ravages of disease, immune suppression does not *cause* disease. Rather, immune suppression is reflective of disease, and so it helps us to gauge the clinical course of disease and the status of our well-being. It plays a part in most every ailment, ranging from the common cold to the emotional state of depression.

The main organs to consider in working with imagery exercises for the immune system are the spleen, the thymus, and the long bones (see diagrams below). The spleen is the seat of humor and laughter. Recall that Norman Cousins, as described in his book *Anatomy of an Illness,* recovered from a life-threatening illness by almost literally laughing himself back to health while watching humorous films that enhanced his immune function.

I have found the following imagery exercise quite helpful in the disease processes that directly affect immune function. I refer to T4 and T8 cells in this exercise. They constitute two major classes of lymphocytes, white blood cells, which are central to the immune system. The T4 cells (also called helper-cells) produce antibodies, which seek out foreign elements in the body and trigger a reaction that leads to the destruction of the invaders. The T8 cells (also called killer-cells) attack invaders directly with potent chemicals.

The Artist of Life

Close your eyes, breathe out three times, and enter your body by any opening you choose, finding your way to the spleen. Breathe out once and see yourself in front of the

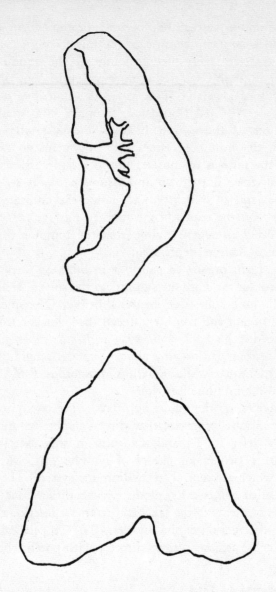

spleen as an artist wearing a beret and holding a palette of paint and brushes. Paint a clown's face on the spleen. See yourself looking at your accomplishment and beginning to smile. As you do, the clown responds by laughing. His mouth opens and his big, long tongue comes out as a river of white lymphocyte cells that you see and sense rushing through your bloodstream to all parts of your body, fighting the illness. See and sense these cells as light, dancing effervescently through your bloodstream, engulfing all foreign invaders. After finishing at the spleen, see yourself traveling up to the thymus. See the thymus as a closed, six-petaled lotus blossom that you gently massage with transparent fingers. As you do, you see the petals open and the T4 immune cell seeds in the center flow out and fly through your body, landing everywhere and planting themselves, reproducing, and fighting and destroying all enemy invaders. See your whole body stimulated and moved at the arrival of these fertile seeds. See and sense the thymus hormone flowing through the now-opened petals and beyond them as a red stream flowing to your long bones, stimulating the bone marrow to produce T4 and T8 white blood cells. See these cells flowing through the blood channels in your bones and acting on your bloodstream. Hear their sound as they call out the enemy invaders from their hiding place in your tissues and organs and destroy them. See, sense, know, and feel the life-giving force furnished you by the movement of these cells. Then open your eyes.

IMPOTENCE

Name: **Saint George Exercise** and **Out of the Maze**
Intention: To restore sexual potency.
Frequency: Once a week on the same morning each week, for 5 to 7 minutes, for three weeks.

Impotence usually refers to a man's inability to have or maintain an erection. Premature ejaculation is sometimes considered a type of impotence. Impotence clearly has an emotional component dealing with inhibitions about sexual matters, which is why it is often called "psychogenic" impotence.

Much has been written about the emotional components of potency problems. For instance, anger experienced toward women, or fear of performing badly, can be associated with impotence. Suffice to say that it can be valuable to investigate the emotional/social issues, as well as the physical ones (mechanical or biological factors), that might be at work in this problem.

Saint George Exercise

Close your eyes. Breathe out twice. See yourself descending into a valley. Meet there a monster or ogre. Have with you whatever you need to fight and defeat this monster. Engage in struggle with the monster, and when you have been victorious and the monster is slain, skin it! Carry the skin with you and ascend from the valley to the top. There, meet your loved one. Take her hand and walk with her to a tree and lie down under it together. See yourselves encased in a cocoon of blue light and embrace. Then open your eyes.

Out of the Maze

Close your eyes. Breathe out three times. See yourself in the center of a labyrinth or maze. While there, imagine the ideal woman, or the woman with whom you are close at present. Find your way out of the labyrinth, paying attention to all turns and all blind alleys. You have to get out to reach this woman. After finding her, take her by the hand to a tree in a meadow. Breathe there in rhythm as part of the universe. See the two of you encased in a blue cocoon. Then kiss and go on sexually, seeing and feeling what happens. Then open your eyes.

INDECISIVENESS

Name: **Scale of Balance** and **The Black Cars**
Intention: To make a decision.
Frequency: As needed, once, for up to 1 minute.

Doubt is the root cause of most all of the bodymind trouble we face in the world. One way this doubt expresses itself frequently is in the vital area of decision-making. Many of you know how painful and never-ending it is to waver over a decision. You find that as you try to "figure out" the answer, no matter how much figuring and added "information" you use, you cannot achieve the certainty you've been looking for—the guarantee that everything will turn out all right. In fact, the more figuring you do, the more the answer seems to recede. In truth, in most cases it is not possible to calculate the right decisions and then to act on them. Decision-making *depends* on a willingness to act, not on an accumulation of more data. Only action gives certainty. One of my favorite imagery exercises for making decisions is **Scale of Balance.** If you are involved with two seemingly equal choices and want to decide between them— two lovers, two job offers, two schools, and so on—try **The Black Cars.**

Scale of Balance

Close your eyes, breathe out three times, and see yourself standing behind a golden balance scale with two golden balance pans. Have with you a pad of white paper. On a slip of paper write an advantage or a positive aspect of one choice and put it on one pan. Continue writing the advantages of this choice, one per slip, and put them in the pan. Then write an advantage or positive aspect of the other choice and put it on the other pan. Again, continue writing the advantages of this choice, one per slip, and put them in the pan. See which pan weighs more, and open your eyes. Then immediately carry out the decision that the pans have indicated.

If the pans remain balanced, look again to see if you have noted and added all the positive advantages of each side of the issue. If the pans still remain balanced, it means either that you are not ready to undertake whatever it is you're concerned with or that you are not as eager to make a change as you think.

The Black Cars

Close your eyes. Breathe out three times and see yourself walking forward down the middle of a one-way, two-lane highway. Two black cars quickly pull up alongside you, one on each side. You spontaneously open the back door of one of the cars and get in. Then look and see who is driving. Open your eyes. Whoever you've seen is the decision you make.

INFERTILITY

Name: **The Fertile Garden**
Intention: To become pregnant.
Frequency: Once a day, for 2 to 3 minutes, for 7 days starting at the beginning of your ovulation, irrespective of how many times you have intercourse.

Infertility can be related to a physical mechanism connected with low hormone production or by a mechanical failure of the ovum to enter the fallopian tube properly. It can also be associated with complex emotional issues. Certainly, ambivalence about having children and feeling tension in the

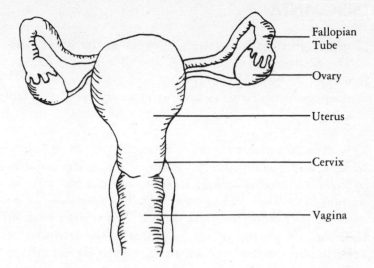

Fallopian
Tube

Ovary

Uterus

Cervix

Vagina

marriage are two issues that can be related to infertility. The following exercise addresses both the physical and psychological aspects.

The Fertile Garden

Close your eyes. Breathe out three times and see yourself going into a beautiful garden. Find there a tree and a stream of flowing water. Bathe in the water, allowing it to enter and to clean all the ova. Come out and sit under a tree with a lot of sun shining through its leaves; the sky is clear blue. Look up to the right and make a wish or prayer for what you want. Do this in an instant. Then call your mate into the garden to join you under the tree. Lie down with him, holding hands. See the blue light forming a dome over you. See what happens with your mate. Afterward, go out of the garden together holding hands, cradling a child between you. Then open your eyes.

INSOMNIA

Name: **Nighttime Reversing, Flowers in the River,** and
   The Setting Sun
Intention: To go to sleep.
Frequency: At bedtime, as long as necessary, until you fall
   asleep.

This sleep disturbance occurs as a difficulty either in falling
asleep or in remaining asleep. There are a couple of pointers
to know about sleep troubles. First, use the bed *only* for
sleeping. Don't eat in bed, read, watch TV, smoke, or do
anything else, other than sleep, in bed. When you are out of
bed, turn on all the lights. Insomnia is the intrusion of
daytime into the sleep period, and since you are not asleep,
make it as much like daytime as possible. When you've had
enough daytime, turn off the lights. The second pointer:
don't fight the thoughts that come. Clear them out by
asking yourself for forgiveness and know that the next day
brings another opportunity to correct your situation. Insomnia represents an inability to forget the day. This inability
frequently has to do with a strong feeling of guilt or weight
of conscience. The fear of death, too, is sometimes expressed
as a sleep disturbance, since sleep can be equated with
death. Often insomnia is noted in depression. Following are
three excellent exercises.

Nighttime Reversing

While lying in bed with your eyes closed, see yourself
going over your day in reverse order, event by event. Start
with the last event of the day and relive it in imagery.
Then, go to the next-to-last and relive it. Go on like this in
reverse order until you reach the point of the day when you
woke up. Go through each event slowly, trying to correct
your attitude and behavior in those situations where you

had difficulty. Also, try to obtain something for yourself that you wanted to get that day but couldn't. If you come across a troubling conversation you had with someone, recall the conversation as close to verbatim as possible—except that now the other person's words come out in your voice and what you said comes out in his or her voice. This experience will relax you, for you will understand what the other person was experiencing (If you wish you might call that person the next day to make amends). Continue this exercise until you fall asleep.

Flowers in the River

While lying in bed with your eyes closed, see yourself lying by the bank of a swiftly flowing river. You are surrounded by flowers. Smell their fragrance. Pick one. Take each preoccupying thought you have, place it in a flower, put the flower in the river, and see and hear it being carried away quickly downstream. Continue this exercise until you fall asleep.

The Setting Sun

Get out of bed. Go to a chair in another room or in another part of the same room. Turn on all the lights. In the chair, close your eyes and see yourself in a meadow where the sun is high in the sky. Lie down, putting your head on a soft tuft of grass, and watch the sun set. See the sun descend slowly below the horizon. When the sun has disappeared and the sky is dark, see yourself leaving the meadow, going to your bed, and sleeping. Then open your eyes, get up from your chair, turn off the lights, and go to bed.

KIDNEY DISTURBANCE

Name: **The Aviary**

Intention: To heal the kidneys.

Frequency: Two or three times a day, for 3 minutes, for 21 days of use and 7 days off. If the problem is not cleared up, use the exercise for two more 21-day cycles with 7 days off in between.

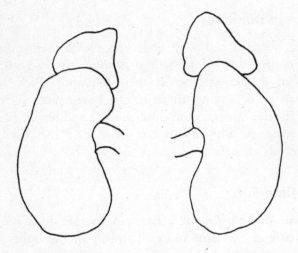

The kidneys are large ear-shaped organs at the area of the left and right flank. Trouble in the kidneys often reflects the inability to make an important decision in your life, or just being chronically indecisive. The more indecisive you are, the more strain you are putting on the kidneys. It can be helpful to use the decision-making exercises (pp. 134–135) for taking care of that problem. For the kidney difficulty itself the following is a helpful exercise.

The Aviary

Close your eyes. Breathe out three times. See yourself in an aviary. The birds are flying freely overhead. Then see, sense, and feel yourself as the mighty ostrich, the bird of the earth. Breathe out once. As the ostrich, imagine yourself forming the largest of its eggs. Sense this egg growing until you gently give it forth into the nest. Sit on it until it becomes the perfect egg. Sense the movement of the yolk and the young bird growing within as the egg grows larger and larger. As it grows, see and know that your kidney(s) is healing. Then open your eyes.

LACK OF VERSION (rotating a fetus)

Name: **Turning the Fetus**
Intention: To turn the fetus in your uterus.
Frequency: When needed, once, for up to 3 minutes. Repeat once if needed.

Version is the medical term for rotating a fetus in the uterus prior to delivery. Medical thinking commonly accepts that the body influences the mental state and emotions—that physical processes create mental effects. This view extends to treatment as well, where drugs not only produce mental effects but are thought to cure emotional disturbances. Logically, it follows that the reverse is true as well—the mental can produce physical changes. I have collected a wealth of clinical instances that demonstrate the immense power that our mental functions have in influencing the body and emotions. In my experience, nowhere has this been more strikingly shown than with two women who succeeded in turning their fetuses using imagery. Both of them were in their eighth month of pregnancy. Each was

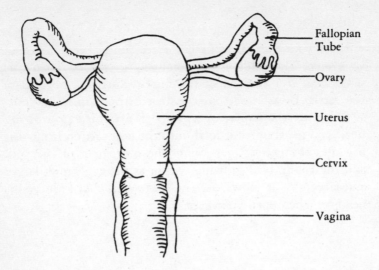

Fallopian
Tube

Ovary

Uterus

Cervix

Vagina

told that she would have a breech delivery and that the fetus could not be turned. With **Turning the Fetus,** they succeeded in doing what presumably could not be done medically. Faith can move fetuses as well as mountains. Don't let anyone tell you different.

Turning the Fetus

Close your eyes. Breathe out three times and enter your body by any opening you choose. Carrying a light with you, find your way to your uterus; *carefully* enter your uterus through the cervix, and find the fetus. Then *carefully* and *very gently* turn the fetus to the proper position, with the head facing down toward the birth canal. Note the sensations, if any, that you experience upon doing so. A sensation of pain, if you have one, will tell you that you are succeeding. Then leave the body by *exactly the way you entered*—back through your uterus and cervix, and out of your body by the entry route. When you are outside of your body, breathe out once and open your eyes. On the next succeeding three days, go back to your uterus and check it to see, imaginally, whether the version (turning) has taken place. Within a week of the exercise, return to your doctor for an examination. If the fetus hasn't turned to the proper delivery position, try the exercise once again—with more conviction this time.

LEUKEMIA

Name: **The Sacred Shadow**
Intention: To heal leukemia.
Frequency: Twice a day, for 1 to 3 minutes, for 7 days.

This cancer of the bone marrow affects young and old alike. Some effective chemotherapy treatments have recently been developed for it, and this form of cancer seems to have a better rate of recovery generally than other forms of cancer.

In my travels I have met two people who independently gave unusual and virtually identical reports about their experience with leukemia. Lying in bed, each saw himself leaving his physical body, and saw this "ethereal" form go to the farthest top corner of the room and tell the physical body lying in the bed that it would be okay and not to worry. The ethereal form then turned upward and asked God for help in healing the body lying in the bed. The ethereal body then returned to the physical body. Within the next 24 to 48 hours, both situations of leukemia cleared up. Soon after, the sister and the wife of a young man in his early thirties who was suffering from acute leukemia came to see me, asking for my help. The man was in a hospital, and the physician working with him had given the family a grave prognosis. I suggested **The Sacred Shadow** exercise to the wife and sister and told them that the entire immediate family should gather in the hospital room and see the man's ethereal body leave his physical body, go to the upper corner of the room, tell him he would be okay, and then turn upward and ask God for help to heal him. They were then to see the ethereal body return to his physical body. The man himself didn't want to participate in this exercise, so he lay there quietly while the family did the imaging around him. Within 24 to 48 hours, the man's condition showed a marked improvement. Within a week, he was discharged from the hospital as recovered.

The Sacred Shadow

Close your eyes and breathe out three times. See your ethereal body leave your physical body and go to an upper corner of the room, where the ceiling meets the walls. Have your ethereal body tell your physical body that everything will be okay. Then have your ethereal body turn upward and ask God to heal your physical body. Afterward, return your ethereal body to your physical body and open your eyes.

LIVER DISTURBANCE

Name: **The Reflecting Mirror**
Intention: To heal the liver.
Frequency: Twice a day, for 1 to 2 minutes, for six 21-day
    cycles of use with 7 days off in between. Check with your
    doctor to see if any improvement has resulted, if the liver
    has reduced in size. Your doctor might want to order a
    standard battery of liver tests to verify your progress. If
    more work is needed, take another three cycles of 21 days
    on, 7 days off.

The liver is the seat of anger (as the heart is the seat of love). The liver has also been recognized as the seat of

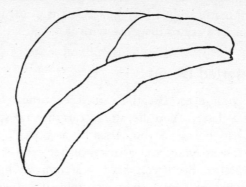

emotion in general. As with anger, forgiveness is a helpful remedy in liver disturbances. When the liver is involved, tell someone you trust about the feelings you are experiencing. The following imagery provides a necessary push toward healing liver disturbances.

The Reflecting Mirror

Close your eyes. Breathe out three times and see your liver as a smooth mirror reflecting your pent-up emotions. Wipe them away to your left with your left hand. Turn the liver over, and on its underside, in the mirror, see your newly reconstructed emotions. Then open your eyes.

LONELINESS

Names: **The Deserted Desert** and **The Deserted Island**
Intention: To overcome loneliness.
Frequency: Twice a day, for up to 5 minutes, for 21 days.

This commonly experienced feeling needs no elaboration except to say that it is associated with staying attached to childhood experiences, not letting go of them so as to enter fully into mature adult life. Loneliness is a real impediment in life, so let's try to dispense with it.

The Deserted Desert

Close your eyes. Breathe out three times. See yourself entering a desert. You are alone, carrying no supplies. See what is happening to you. Breathe out once. See a figure coming toward you from a distance; see who it is as he or she approaches. See if you want to accompany him or her or if you prefer to continue by yourself. If you go with the figure, what advice does he or she give you? Otherwise, go on by yourself until you want to turn back and return by the same route. If you go with the figure and get advice, then you should also return by the same route. As you return, know that your loneliness has gone. Then open your eyes.

The Deserted Island

Close your eyes. Breathe out three times and find yourself alone on a deserted, desolate island. You have with you a shirt or cloth, which you attach to the top of a very high tree to signal a passing ship or plane. See what you do on your journey around the island. After you finish, see that a boat or plane comes. See your return to civilization—your trip from the island to the plane or boat, and then on back to your home. As you return, know that your loneliness has disappeared. Then open your eyes.

MONONUCLEOSIS

Name: **The White Knights, The Intimate Defender,** and **The White Eagle** (all are useful for stimulating the immune system)
Intention: To be free of mononucleosis.
Frequency: Once a day, for 3 minutes, for 7 days for each exercise—a total of 21 days.

Mononucleosis, the "kissing sickness," is characterized by bouts of unusual tiredness and fatigue for no apparent reason. Varying periods of debilitation are also associated with it. Mononucleosis seems to be transmitted primarily through kissing, hence the popular nickname. It also occurs more commonly in young people, and it mimics many other, more serious illnesses, often being the first diagnosis after everything else has been ruled out. There has been no definitive medical treatment discovered for this ailment, except for several weeks of bed rest. The following treatment regimen should be performed over a three-week period.

The White Knights—Week 1

Close your eyes. Breathe out three times. The white knights have to fight an army of warriors occupying a fortified place. After pushing out the warriors, the knights must fight them off once again during a counterattack the warriors mount in an effort to retake the fort. Then open your eyes.

The Intimate Defender—Week 2

Close your eyes. Breathe out three times. See the white spots of a leopard's skin. See yourself entering the skin of the great, white-spotted leopard; your hands and feet are completely covered by the skin. (Those of you who have had an operation or injury can see the organ or area returning to its original unscarred form.) See, sense, repair, and put in perfect order all the white spots that are not perfect. Make them all perfectly white and round by planting white hair all around to make a perfect form. When your leopard skin is perfect, feel yourself perfectly well and emerge from it slowly. Then open your eyes.

The White Eagle—Week 3

Close your eyes. Breathe out three times. Be a white eagle in the sky. Spot a movement on the ground and know that it is a jaguar. Swoop down and kill the young jaguar and fly back to your nest with it as food for your eaglets. Then spot two young jaguars on the ground. Swoop down, and with each talon take the jaguars back to the nest. Each day repeat, taking two jaguars back to the nest as food. Then open your eyes.

MULTIPLE SCLEROSIS

Name: **Ladder of Lights**
Intention: To heal the nervous system.
Frequency: Every 2 to 3 hours while awake, for nine cycles of 21 days of use and 7 days off. During each cycle, in the first week do the exercise for 2 to 3 minutes; in the second week, for 1 to 2 minutes; in the third week, for 30 seconds.

This imagery exercise is an example of how imagery techniques may affect the nervous system in general. When your nervous system has been damaged, usually only part of the system is damaged, so that some part is still functioning. This functioning part must be stimulated through imagery, for the movement promoted there will promote movement in the damaged part. There is a relay mechanism in the nervous system by which impulses are passed from above to below, and vice versa, as well as from right to left and vice versa. The stimulation through imagery can come, for example, from light aimed at the nerve, thereby evoking some feeling or sensation. Of course, other sorts of imaginal stimuli can be used as well. Do not give up hope, and don't believe that paralysis is a hopeless condition to overcome.

The key in focusing imagery exercises for nervous system damage is the above-below, right-left axes of the body. For example, if a patient has nerve damage in the right leg, we would work on the healthy nerves in the left forearm. The leg below is mirrored by the forearm above on the opposite side—above-below, right-left. The diaphragm is the dividing point. If you lay the upper part of the body on the lower part, using the diaphragm as the median point, there is almost perfect symmetry. For instance, the fingers and toes match, as wrists and ankles, elbows and knees, shoulders and hips, and so on. Keep this organization of above-below and right-left in mind when you consider imagery for a damaged nervous system.

Following is a specific imagery exercise for multiple sclerosis. It is important to know that in multiple sclerosis, white blood cells, which will attack any substance perceived as an invader, misperceive as an enemy the myelin sheath covering nerves, and so they mistakenly attack and destroy it.

Ladder of Lights

Close your eyes. Breathe out three times. Demand inwardly that your body (and any medication that you are taking) produce all its healing substances. Sense and feel the substances being released. Breathe out once and see all the nerve cells being fed these healing substances. Breathe out once and see and sense the suppressor T-cells—a type of white blood cell directly involved in immune function—teaching the other white blood cells to distinguish friends

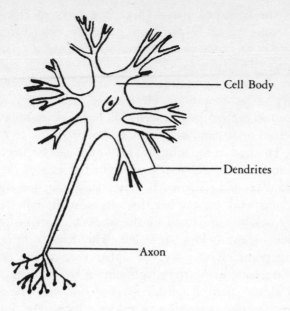

(the myelin sheath) from foe (bacteria). Sense and see this happening all along the spinal column, from the bottom to the top and up into the brain, as a ladder of flashing lights sending sparks of electrical energy throughout the body. Breathe out once and see and sense the nerves being remyelinated from the brain down to the bottom of the spinal column, seeing the energy streaming down as golden white spiral cascades. Then open your eyes.

MUSCLE SPASM

Name: **Transparent Fingers** and **The Ice Exercise**
Intention: To relieve muscle spasm.
Frequency: As needed every 15 to 30 minutes, for 2 to 3 minutes, until spasm is gone.

Tightness and spasm of muscles occur often and with regularity in many people for a variety of reasons that can be mechanical or emotional in nature. You should look to see if any emotional circumstance or social situation was going on when the spasm occurred. Whatever the reason, the spasm must be attended to immediately. Following are two quick ways to do so.

Transparent Fingers

Close your eyes. Breathe out three times and begin, in your imagery, to massage your muscle with your transparent fingers. As you do so, sense the blood flowing through the muscle and see the muscle filling with light from above. While massaging, see the muscle elongating as you tease apart the strands and release the knots. Know that when the light has filled the muscle, the blood is flowing through it freely, the muscle is long and unknotted, and the spasm has gone. Then open your eyes.

The Ice Exercise

Close your eyes. Breathe out three times and see your muscle encased in a block of ice. See the ice melting, knowing that as it melts, the muscle is relaxing. After the ice has completely melted, open your eyes, knowing that the spasm has gone.

OBESITY

Name: **Mirroring Yourself**
Intention: To lose weight, to become thin.
Frequency: As needed when you want to lose weight, for 1 to 2 minutes.

Name: **Restructuring the Body**

Intention: To lose weight, to become thin.

Frequency: 20 to 30 minutes before each meal, for up to 1 minute, for three cycles of 21 days of use and 7 days off in between. During the second and third cycles, you also apply the exercise just as you are ready to eat. You can stop the exercise as soon as you achieve your desired outcome.

It seems there are many emotional matters interwoven in the obesity problem. This problem is experienced as muted unhappiness connected with beliefs about scarcity in your life. Survival is an "issue" here, for you believe that scarcity could lead to starvation and death. You feel deprived of nourishment and don't make your needs known openly. You react to this by overeating.

Your own effort is the key factor to the success of any weight-loss regimen. This imagery exercise should help you sort out the emotional correlates of your dissatisfaction with your weight.

These exercises may be used along with other weight-loss regimens you might be employing, or you may use them on their own, especially if all else has failed.

Mirroring Yourself

One important aspect in weight loss is to maintain some image of who/what you would like to look like when the weight is lost.

Imagine yourself in a mirror, seeing yourself thinner there and then seeing yourself enter the mirror and merging with this image. Notice the sensations you experience. Come out of the mirror, stand in front of it again, and push the image out of the mirror to the right with your right hand. Each time you sit down to eat, or several minutes beforehand, see this image you're becoming. You might like to draw this image on a sheet of paper and hang it where you can see it frequently. You might even like to take it with you if you are away from home for long periods of time. Seeing this picture for a moment reinforces your intention.

Restructuring the Body

The purpose of this exercise is to shift the emphasis from weight loss to altering the shape of your body. When you restructure, you commonly lose weight as well. Draw a picture of yourself, labeling in inches the parts of your body you would like to change.

About 20 to 30 minutes before eating, sit in a chair and imagine all four extremities folding in. See the fingers and toes fold into the hands and feet; folding into the wrists and ankles; folding into the forearms and elbows and calves and knees; folding into the upper arms and shoulders and thighs and hips; all folding into the abdomen under the diaphragm and meeting there. This should be done while quickly inhaling one deep breath. On the outbreath, see gray smoke coming out and drifting away in the air. Do this exercise three times, as quickly as it takes you to inhale. Afterward, get up from the chair and stand by a wall. Facing north, stretch up on your toes and stretch your arms in the air. Then make a quarter turn to the right, stretch again on your toes, and stretch your right arm. Make another quarter turn and stretch on the toes, and stretch both arms. Make another quarter turn, stretch on the toes, and stretch the left arm. Repeat this process twice more. Do this exercise for one week.

In the second week, continue the first week's exercise and add the following: when you sit down to eat, tell yourself the content of your meal that you are about to eat. Then tell your body to take in exactly what it needs and to reject what it doesn't need. Do this at every meal for the next two weeks.

During the third week, add the following: 20 to 30

minutes before eating, after completing the folding and stretching exercise, sit back in the chair, close your eyes, breathe in, and physically bend your body over from the waist, elevating your legs and stretching them while stretching your arms straight out in front of you. On the exhalation, see your arms and legs extending far, far out in front of you and touching a structure at some great distance from you—for example, sitting in New York City, see your extremities stretching across the Hudson River, touching against some building on the New Jersey side. Then relax. Repeat this part of the exercise another two times.

After week three, stop the exercises for 7 days and measure the parts you have wanted to change. If you have not succeeded then repeat this series for two more cycles of 21 days on and 7 days off. Carry on this work thereafter, if needed, for as many cycles as you need for a successful outcome.

OBSESSIVE THOUGHTS

Names: **Thought for Food** and **Lightswitch**
Intention: To control excessive thinking.
Frequency: Daily as needed, for a few seconds.

Some of us cannot control the outpourings of our mind, and we find ourselves in the grip of a seemingly endless deluge of thoughts that are distracting, deceptive, and downright disturbing. In psychological terminology, this situation is called "obsessional" thinking. It's as though some little demon got in there and took over the controls of the thinking ship. Following are two imagery exercises that can help you regain control of the ship. Please note that neither of these exercises requires any special breathing out when using them.

Thought for Food

Close your eyes. See each thought as a worm. Feed the worm to a bird that comes and flies off with it. Do it quickly. Then open your eyes.

Lightswitch

Close your eyes. See a red lightswitch in your left cerebral hemisphere. Shut off the switch to stop your thoughts. Then open your eyes.

PAIN

Name: **Painless Voyage**
Intention: To stop pain.
Frequency: Every 10 to 15 minutes, for 3 to 5 minutes, until pain subsides.

Name: **Befriending Pain**
Intention: To stop pain.
Frequency: Every 10 to 15 minutes, for 2 to 3 minutes, until pain subsides.

Name: **Through the Magnifying Glass, Handling Pain, and The Helping Bird**
Intention: To stop pain.
Frequency: Every 10 to 15 minutes, for 1 to 2 minutes, until pain subsides.

Name: **Rockets into Space**
Intention: To stop head pain.
Frequency: Every 10 to 15 minutes, for 1 to 2 minutes, until pain subsides.

Name: **Emptying the Socket**
Intention: To stop tooth pain.
Frequency: Every 5 minutes, for 1 to 2 minutes, until pain
　subsides.

Pain is an important mechanism for our bodily functioning.
It alerts us to the presence of some trouble. In this sense, it
is not only an "adversary," an enemy that we believe must be
stopped at all costs, but also a messenger, a teacher of sorts,
signaling some danger. In English the root of the word *pain*
means "punishment"; in Sanskrit, it means "purification."

As I explained earlier, when you ask yourself for an image
to express an emotion or sensation, the image usually comes
quickly. Nowhere is this fact more evident than when
working with pain.

I include here five exercises for pain in general, one for
head pain, and one for tooth pain. (In the case of tooth
pain, you should consult your dentist to determine the source
of the pain. If your head pain persists, see your doctor.)

Find the exercise, or a combination of them, that brings
you relief. After doing them, give yourself time to see if the
pain has disappeared. Take 5 or 10 minutes to gauge it.
Amidst all this, do try to find some meaning for the pain.
Is there a punishment, some guilt, some message? For the
tooth pain, try to find any current acute loss you may be
suffering from. If you don't find something, you can still
work on eliminating pain. If you find something, then an
additional learning experience can take place. Acknowledge
these messages and face them directly. You may immediately realize that some decision or action in your life has to
be taken. Don't hesitate to do so.

Painless Voyage

Close your eyes. Breathe out one time. See the pain.
After seeing it, find yourself entering your body with a gold
can of hot, golden oil. Make your way to the pain. Have a

light with you and examine the pain from every angle. Then pour the hot, golden oil over the pain, covering it completely. See the pain dissolve to a golden point. Turn around and see golden rays of health and well-being flowing from this point to all parts of the body. Then leave your body by the route you entered, knowing that your pain has gone. Then open your eyes.

Befriending Pain

Close your eyes. Breathe out one time. See the pain. After seeing it, know that you can befriend it by entering into it and sit in the center of it. Stay there and don't complain about it. (By "complain," I mean *not* giving it such attributes as "awful," "terrible," "horrible"; in other words, don't give it any negative adjectival labels.) Then open your eyes.

Through the Magnifying Glass

Close your eyes. Breathe out once. See your pain. Look at it from every angle through a magnifying glass, then erase it by wiping it away to the left. Then open your eyes.

Handling Pain

Close your eyes. Breathe out once. See yourself with very big, strong hands. With your two big hands remove the pain and throw it away. Then open your eyes.

The Helping Bird

Close your eyes. Breathe out three times. Look at a bird. Ask him to take away your pain. See him pecking at it with his beak and flying away with the pieces. When all the pieces are gone, open your eyes.

Rockets into Space (for head pain)

Close your eyes. Breathe out three times and see yourself putting the points of pain on rockets shooting out of your head and disappearing into space. Then open your eyes.

Emptying the Socket (for tooth pain)

Close your eyes and breathe out three times. See yourself gently pushing out your tooth (use any degree of vigor you wish to remove the tooth). Breathe out once and feel air coming into the opening, where a little of the gum and nerve are showing. Breathe out once and put the tooth back lightly into place, knowing that it is healthy and whole. Breathe out once, and see the swelling going down as you breathe out three times. Then open your eyes.

PANCREATITIS

Name: **The Healing Rainbow**
Intention: To heal the pancreas, to bring it back to harmonious functioning.
Frequency: Four times a day, for up to 3 minutes, for 21 days.

Name: **Correcting Cruelty**
Intention: To heal the pancreas.
Frequency: Three times a day, for 2 to 3 minutes, for 21 days.

Inflammation of the pancreas is called "pancreatitis." The name is somewhat misleading because this inflammation does not begin directly with the pancreas but is usually found to occur secondarily in association with acute or chronic

alcohol intoxication, biliary tract disturbances, or for unknown reasons. Alcohol not only affects the liver but devas-
tates the pancreas. Following are short imagery exercises
that can help alleviate the symptoms and promote healing.
If you are receiving medical treatment for pancreatitis, these
exercises are excellent in conjunction with the treatment. It
may be helpful to know that the pancreas often has to do
with cruelty directed either against ourselves or against
someone else.

The Healing Rainbow

Close your eyes. Breathe out three times. See yourself
entering your body by any opening that you choose and find
your way to your pancreas. Have a light with you and
examine your pancreas from every angle. Next, see yourself
weaving a rainbow of lights around your pancreas. See and
know that this rainbow is at first surrounding your pancreas
and then is penetrating directly into it, quieting it, repairing its walls, and eliminating pain. Then open your eyes.

Correcting Cruelty

Close your eyes. Breathe out three times. See, sense, and
know the cruelty experienced by your pancreas. Do what is
necessary to correct this cruelty, seeing your pancreas becoming pale yellow as it heals. Then open your eyes.

PANIC

Name: **No Limits**
Intention: To stop panic.
Frequency: As needed every 5 to 10 minutes, for 1 minute.

Name: **The Coffin of Cure** and **The Pan Exercise**
Intention: To stop panic.
Frequency: As needed every 1 to 2 hours, for 3 minutes, until panic subsides.

This emotional reaction disables many people. It effectively paralyzes action, giving you the sense that you are falling apart and that any movement you make will result only in worse chaos for you. It is an overpowering feeling of terror. There is often a strong feeling of loneliness preceding the panic attack, the sudden realization of which often elicits the episode. If you are subject to such attacks, it would be worthwhile to review the imagery exercises for loneliness (p. 145). Following are some possibilities for you to try at the outset, or even during the experience.

Find the exercise or combination of exercises that works for you. I've found that humor is an excellent antidote in helping to calm the panic response.

No Limits

Close your eyes. Breathe out three times *very slowly*. See, sense, feel, and know that your body has no biological limits. Keep the experience for a *long* moment. Then open your eyes, knowing that your panic has disappeared.

The Coffin of Cure

Close your eyes. Breathe out three times *very slowly*. You are in a coffin wrapped as a mummy. The lid is closed.

Accept your feelings. Stay with them for a *long* moment. Push open the lid, step out, and unwrap the bandages, making a ball out of them. Throw the ball into a dark cloud that has formed overhead, seeing it go to the center, breaking up the cloud. Let the rainwater wash over you, knowing your panic has gone. See how the landscape looks before opening your eyes.

The Pan Exercise

Close your eyes. Breathe out three times *very slowly*. See the god Pan playing his pipes, and the children following him into a *seemingly* lovely place at the edge of a cliff. Choose not to be lured and not to enter this procession. Breathe out once. Turn around and find your way to the center of a clearing. Build a fence around this clearing. Decide who can enter. Know that your panic has now been restrained. Then open your eyes.

POLYPS AND TUMORS
(see also **Breast Cysts**)

Name: **Cell of the Universe**
Intention: To shrink the tumor (in this case, polyp).
Frequency: Twice a day, for 1 to 3 minutes, for 21 days. After this time, have the tumor examined again by your doctor. If you require further work, use this imagery for two more 21-day cycles with 7 days off between them. During the 7 days off, if you should think of your polyp, think of it as gone.

Name: **The Healing Laser**
Intention: To shrink the tumor (in this case, fibroids).
Frequency: Three times a day, for 2 to 3 minutes, for three cycles of 21 days of use and 7 days off.

There are various sorts of benign tumors that occur anywhere in the body. They can appear as cysts, fatty tumors, or any of a variety of solid tumors of muscle, and even as polyps. Generally, any tumorous growth, no matter where it shows up, alerts us to some imbalance in our lives on all levels. My personal belief is that when we correct the imbalance, the tumorous growth clears up! I've had patients with cysts, fibroid tumors, polyps, and the like, who have dealt with them quite well through imagery. One middle-aged woman had had a chronic polyp in her left nostril for most of her adult life. It contributed in no small measure to a longstanding asthmatic condition. She told me that she had not been able to breathe through her left nostril for as long as she could remember and had been to many "breathing specialists" to no avail. In connection with our work on her asthma, she also focused on the polyp that had effectively closed her left nostril. She used **The Cell of the Universe** exercise, and her polyp receded so that she could breathe normally through her left nostril.

A second patient, a woman with several uterine fibroid tumors, decided to try imagery before submitting herself to the surgery recommended by her gynecologist. After three cycles of **The Healing Laser**, she didn't require surgery or any further visits to the gynecologist for this condition.

The Cell of the Universe

Close your eyes. Breathe out three times. See and sense your polyp contracting to a single cell. Sense all the material being expressed and sense the dryness of the cell. See yourself sitting inside the cell and know this dryness. Then break through the membrane at any part of the cell, take the fragmented pieces in your hand, and offer them as a gift to the universe. Then open your eyes.

The Healing Laser

Close your eyes. Breathe out three times. See yourself entering your body by any opening you choose. Take a light with you. Find your way to your uterus and examine the fibroids to determine their location, size, and color. Bring a tube of blue laser light and focus it directly at the fibroids, seeing them shrink and shrivel up, then direct a tube of golden laser light around the base of the fibroids and laser-surgically excise the fibroids that remained after using the blue laser light. See the golden laser cut in a circular motion around the base of these now shrunken growths, and then remove them by hand. Then find the right color laser tube to promote the growth of healthy cells there and see the whole area heal up and look exactly like the surrounding healthy tissue. After the normal cells are stimulated and healing takes place, leave your body via the route by which you entered. Once outside your body, breathe out and open your eyes.

POSTURAL DISTURBANCE

Name: **Standing Tall**
Intention: To straighten posture.
Frequency: As often as you can remember to do it, the first
    several times for 1 to 2 minutes, thereafter, for an instant
    whenever you think of it.

Almost everyone is concerned about standing tall, for one's posture very clearly denotes one's state of mind. When things are "weighing" us down, or we feel a sense of inferiority or alienation, we tend to slump or slouch. Standing erect imparts an air of confidence. Another benefit of straight posture is that we breathe better, which is of great importance for our health. Following is a simple but extremely effective imagery exercise for establishing straight posture. Once you know how to do it, you can do it anywhere, with your eyes open. By constant repetition you can reeducate your body to a different posture.

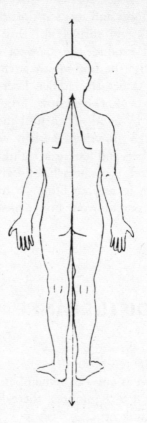

Standing Tall

Close your eyes. Breathe out once and see a silver cord spring from the top of your head straight up into the sky. At the same time, see a silver cord running from the base of your skull straight down the center of your back, between your legs, and going directly into the earth. Simultaneously, see a silver cord running from the tip of each wing (scapula) of the back at an angle up to, and joining, the cord at the base of the skull. Imagine all four cords pulling at the same moment. See how you look and feel. Then open your eyes.

Whenever you do this exercise, with your eyes open or closed, see the silver cords and experience the four pulls for an instant, then see how you look and feel, knowing that you are standing perfectly straight.

PREMENSTRUAL SYNDROME
(see also **Swelling**)

Name: **The Desert Sand**
Intention: To eliminate bloating.
Frequency: From the first sight of premenstrual symptoms
    to the end of menstruation, three to four times a day, for
    1 to 2 minutes.

Millions of women suffer from irritability, bloating, depression, pain, and numerous other symptoms usually beginning 7 to 10 days before menstruation. Several physiological changes are taking place, the most prominent of which are water retention, which leads to bloating, and calcium loss, which is involved in the emotional disturbances experienced at this time. The following imagery exercise may be quite useful in reducing or eliminating the bloating and, in helping, may make this premenstrual time much easier to navigate. (Also taking calcium supplementation may be quite helpful in eliminating the emotional distress. You should ask a health professional to recommend dosages.)

The Desert Sand

Close your eyes and breathe out three times. See yourself in a desert. Cover your body with sand. Have the sun bake it into your skin. *Sense* the sand soaking up your internal water and the sun drying up the sand. Then open your eyes.

PREPARING YOURSELF FOR SURGERY

Name: **Coming Through Surgery**
Intention: To come through surgery in good shape.
Frequency: Every morning, for 1 to 2 minutes, for the 7 days preceding the operation.

Going into the hospital for an operation, no matter how "minor" the procedure is thought to be, often instills a sense of anxiety. Following is a simple way to manage any upcoming surgery.

Coming Through Surgery

Close your eyes. Breathe out once and see yourself *after* the operation, sitting up in bed, smiling, and receiving visitors. Then see yourself getting dressed and walking out of the hospital, hand in hand with your loved one, going out the front door and either walking or driving home. Then open your eyes.

PROSTATE ENLARGEMENT

Name: **The Golden Net**
Intention: To reduce prostate enlargement.
Frequency: Twice a day, for 3 to 5 minutes, for six cycles of
21 days of use with 7 days off in between.

This most common ailment among older males has resulted
in much long-term suffering, not only for the symptoms it
can cause, such as urinary retention, but for the many
postoperative disturbances that can occur. One of the most
common of these is depression. In my practice, I have seen a
number of instances where prostate enlargement has arisen
in connection with sexual disturbances ranging from chronic
masturbation, to prior venereal infection, to extramarital
affairs with attendant guilt feelings long unexpressed. Long
unhappy relationships, in which the unhappiness is not
expressed, also seem to affect this organ. We might say that
an enlarged prostate in many instances equals unhappiness.

As you employ this exercise, understand that it can be
valuable for you to tell yourself that you've made an error in
behavior and to ask yourself for forgiveness. The following
example shows how important this is.

A man in his late fifties came to see me because he
was suffering from an enlarged prostate with attendant
symptoms of urinary retention and difficulty initiating the
urinary stream. He had been told by his physician that
he would require an operation, but wanted to try imagery
first.

In the course of the treatment, during which I saw this
patient once a week, he very quickly was able to identify an
important problematic area in his life that he related to his
malfunctioning prostate. Fortunately, he was able to correct
this problematic situation in his life. Six months later, his
family doctor examined him and discovered that the prostate was of normal size and no longer required surgery. A

two-year follow-up revealed no significant change in his prostate, and his overall life functioning had also markedly improved.

The Golden Net

Close your eyes. Breathe out three times and see yourself entering your body by any opening you choose and finding your prostate. When you have done this, examine it from every angle. Then see yourself placing a thin golden net encircling the prostate. The net has a drawstring that you must pull around your prostate as tightly as you can stand, as you see the gland reducing to its normal size. Then, using your other hand, gently massage the prostate, sensing the seminal fluid and/or urine flowing smoothly and evenly through the neck of the bladder into the urethra, and down the urethra to the tip of the penis, from which you see the fluid flowing in a stream into the earth, at the same time seeing your prostate shrinking to its normal size. Then open your eyes.

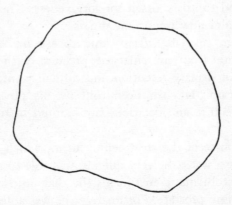

PSORIASIS

Name: **Arctic Scaling**

Intention: To clear up psoriasis.

Frequency: Three cycles of 21 days on and 7 days off for 3 minutes for the first cycle, then 1 to 2 minutes for the second and 30 seconds to 1 minute for the third. If by then it hasn't cleared up or improved, consult your doctor. If it has begun to clear, but not completely, use as many cycles of imagery as you need to heal.

Psoriasis is a common skin disease affecting up to 4 percent of the white population (very few blacks are affected). It can be confined to a local area or can be widespread covering the entire body. A disabling form of arthritis can occur with this ailment. Emotional and social factors are prominent in this condition as we might expect. Very often there are mixed feelings of anger and grief combining in a context of severe turmoil, confusion, and frustration about social relationships. Many of these feelings go into a "deep freeze" in the psoriasis sufferer. It is this "deep freeze" experience that gives rise to the psoriasis exercise to be described below called **Arctic Scaling**.

"Greg" was a young man who had developed psoriasis four years before arriving at my office covered from head to toe with psoriatic scales and showing the possible beginnings of arthritic changes in his fingers. He had been on practically all of the latest psoriatic treatment regimens without any improvement. Using imagery was for Greg a last resort before turning to the remaining severe medical treatments left to him—some of which are toxic and others of which may increase the likelihood of skin cancer—which he wanted to avoid.

Greg used two imagery exercises: **Arctic Scaling** and the **Inside-Outside** exercise used for the gastrointestinal tract. This latter one was introduced because in my understanding of psoriasis there is a relationship between this condition and toxic buildup in the colon—his diet was high in fat and he tended to consume a great deal of "fast food" meals. I spoke to him three months later, after he had completed three cycles of imagery activity. He had become more careful about his diet, had not taken any medication, and had performed the two imagery exercises faithfully. The result was that the psoriasis had almost completely cleared up 90%; he had only a few spots left. He said there was "no doubt" that the imagery did the job. Here is the **Arctic Scaling** exercise that he used:

Arctic Scaling

Close your eyes. Breathe out three times. See, sense, and feel yourself naked. You are sitting at the North Pole. You have with you a golden ice pick with which you remove all the white scales on your body until you see the healthy skin underneath. After you have shed the scales, go into the cold, Arctic water, sensing and feeling it washing your skin thoroughly. Then come out of the water and see and sense an icy film of Arctic water covering your entire body. Have a jar of golden whale oil with which you cover your entire body over the icy film of water. Put on a royal purple gown or robe as you see your body healthy and free of scales. Then open your eyes.

RESPIRATORY DISEASE
(see also **Breathing Problems**)

Name: **Airing the House**
Intention: To breathe normally.
Frequency: Every hour, for 1 to 2 minutes, daily till breathing normalizes.

Name: **Egyptian Temple**
Intention: To breathe normally, to heal the lungs.
Frequency: Four times a day, for 3 minutes, for three cycles
    of 21 days of use with 7 days off in between.

Name: **The Bellows**
Intention: To breathe normally.
Frequency: Six times at the first sitting, then six times every
    30 minutes for 1 hour, so that you've done this exercise
    eighteen times in 60 minutes. Then, 6 hours later, do
    the same thing; and again 6 hours later. Do each bellows
    movement for 15 to 30 seconds, for 21 days.

Many of us suffer from some sort of respiratory discomfort.
Instead of detailing them all, I will give you a couple of
strong exercises that can be applied to the problem in general.
Breathing is a matter of "life and breath"—read *death*—
as the advertisements say. Breathing problems are statements
of our experience of many life situations—constriction versus
freedom, life versus death, crying versus joy. Some of us
want to know what our last breath will be like, concerned
as we are deep down with what death is about, yet we will
naturally gasp for air if we feel breath leaving us. I raise
this point because we may be, or may know, people who
would rather die than give up smoking as we (they) wheeze
with emphysema (chronic respiratory constriction, with
resultant inelasticity of the lungs). Here is a perfect example
of the tension going on between wanting to live and wanting
to die. At any rate, these breath exercises are helpful, and
you might also refer to those I've prescribed for asthma.

    If you want to improve your overall breathing capacity,
irrespective of any disturbance, try the following: Breathe
from 5 to 1, counting each inhalation as a number. Then
inhale once more, going from 1 to 0, and see the zero
becoming yourself. Then breathe out from 1 to 5, each
outbreath being a new number, feeling yourself expanding
more with each number.

The following exercises can be done singly or in any combination you wish.

Airing the House

Close your eyes. Breathe out three times. See your body as a house that has windows. Each cycle of breathing is the opening of the windows one by one, and you are breathing in fresh air. After the last window has been opened, open your eyes.

Egyptian Temple

Close your eyes. Breathe out three times. See, sense, and feel yourself entering an ancient Egyptian temple. Know that the inside is constructed according to the plan of the human body. Greet the keeper at the entrance. Let him or her take you to the chamber of the chest. See yourself in a long hallway with a large room on either side. See the rooms fill completely with light from above. Sense and feel what happens in your lungs. Thank the keeper as he or she

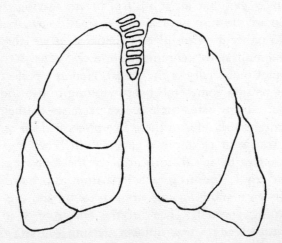

takes you back to the entrance, and say good-bye. Make the journey in slowly and exit more quickly. After finishing, open your eyes.

The Bellows

Close your eyes. Breathe out once. See your lungs as a pair of bellows. As you breathe in, the bellows expand. See and sense the lungs expanding to the width of the chest. As you breathe out, the bellows close, expelling the air forcibly. Then open your eyes.

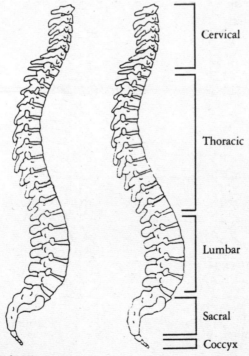

Side View

Cervical

Thoracic

Lumbar

Sacral

Coccyx

SCOLIOSIS (curvature of the spine)

Name: **Seeing Straight**
Intention: To correct curvature of the spine.
Frequency: As often as you remember, for 1 second, until
the curvature corrects.

Curvature of the spine is found in a large segment of the
population. It begins in early childhood, has no known
cause within medical circles, and is seen in medicine as
merely a part of the body's growth process. However, I
believe this condition has to do with a statement the person

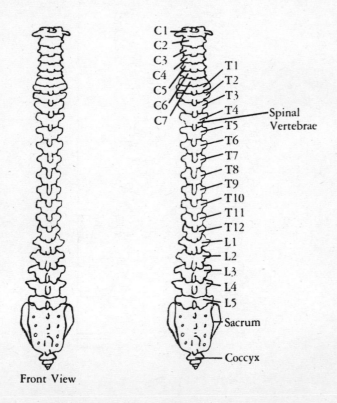

C1
C2
C3
C4
C5
C6
C7

T1
T2
T3
T4
T5
T6
T7
T8
T9
T10
T11
T12

Spinal
Vertebrae

L1
L2
L3
L4
L5

Sacrum

Coccyx

Front View

is making about his or her stunted growth. This curvature may become more and more severe as the years go on. We can see the effects of this condition in a process known as "hunchback," where the curvature of the dorsal vertebrae is exaggerated; or in a process known as "lordosis," where the lumbar curvature is exaggerated. The imagery that can bring about correction is relatively simple to do.

Seeing Straight

See and sense for an instant, *anytime* you remember to do so, your spinal column in its normal curvature—as drawn in the diagram. You may have your eyes open or closed as you wish.

SELF-DOUBT

Name: **Be Your Own Hero**
Intention: To bolster self-esteem or self-confidence.
Frequency: Twice a day, for 1 to 2 minutes, for 21 days.

If, unfortunately, you are unwittingly down on yourself, I would bet it is because you are comparing yourself to someone else. This is a very serious mistake. You don't yet realize that you are incomparable. There is no one like you in the entire world, not even your identical twin. The following exercise is quite simple. See what happens to you in the three-week period you use it.

Be Your Own Hero

Close your eyes. Breathe out three times. Be your own hero. Acting as your own hero, overcome all the obstacles in your life. Then open your eyes.

SEPARATED SHOULDER

Name: **Locating the Shoulder**
Intention: To put your shoulder back in place.
Frequency: As needed for 30 seconds.

Many people experience spontaneous dislocations of joints, particularly the shoulder. Often these dislocations occur as a result of strenuous athletic activity. It's helpful to understand the meaning of the shoulder, clearly spelled out in such common phrases as "shouldering responsibility," "he's got the weight of the world on his shoulders," "shouldering the burden," and so on. Sometimes the burdens become too great to bear and the shoulders give way.

I was riding the subway one day. I met an acquaintance there, a young man in his early twenties. As we were talking, I sitting down, he standing up holding on to a strap, he suddenly screamed out in pain and fell to the floor, writhing in obvious agony. He told me that his shoulder chronically became dislocated, and it could happen anytime, anywhere. I instructed him in the **Locating the Shoulder** exercise. After finishing the exercise, he blinked several times, moved his arm normally, found the pain had gone, and thanked me profusely.

Locating the Shoulder

When the dislocation occurs and you are able to be quiet enough to allow yourself to image, close your eyes and see your shoulder slipping easily back into the shoulder joint and see your arm then hanging normally. After going through the imagery, immediately put the shoulder back in place physically. You can do this yourself or you can have someone else who is familiar with this problem do it—but only *after* the imagery exercise.

SKIN DISORDERS
(see also **Acne**)

Name: **Egyptian Healing**
Intention: To clear up your skin.
Frequency: Three times a day, for 3 to 4 minutes, for 21
days.

For general skin disorders, there is one excellent imagery
exercise outlined below. First, however, I want to make
several points concerning the skin and imagery from a
physical and emotional perspective. I think it is fairly
evident that emotions play a prominent role in skin problems. Such phrases as "thin skinned," "skin deep," and
"thick skinned" attest to the connection between emotions
and skin. When rashes break out, they are referred to as
"eruptions," and when we are angry, our skin often erupts.
The same thing happens if we are frightened. Anger eruptions are usually red, while fright eruptions are white, like
goosebumps. Needless to say, there are many positive feelings associated with skin sensations, loving and sexual ones
most significantly.

In terms of the physical component of skin disorders,
imagery works with colors. To understand what color to use
may require trial and error, but once you apply a color, you
will know right away whether it is working. As a general
rule, it is wise to use the color that neutralizes the one that
is involved in the disturbance. Many rashes and inflamma-
tions are red; therefore, *blue* is usually effective, since blue
neutralizes red. Rashes are also classified as either dry or
oily, so the healing process uses drying imagery for oily
rash, and oily imagery for dry rash. For example, an oozing
rash may be dried by using sunlight; a dry, scaly rash may
be helped by using the oil of a coconut palm leaf.

The general imagery exercise is the **Egyptian Healing**,
with specific directions for use on the skin.

Egyptian Healing

Follow the directions for **Egyptian Healing** on p. 45 to the point where the sun's rays come into your palms and extend beyond each fingertip, and at the end of each ray of each fingertip of your right hand is a complete small hand, while at the end of each ray of each fingertip of your left hand is an eye. (If you are left-handed, the small hands and the eyes should be reversed.) Now, turn these rays to your skin, knowing that the eyes emit light and can also see. Using them, look at the skin area that is bothering you. In one of the small hands have a golden brush with fine golden bristles. With it clean off the area thoroughly till the affected area is free of all rash, and clean skin can be seen underneath. In another small hand hold a tube of blue light that emerges as a laser light, which you shine directly on the area that has been cleaned in order to promote healing by stimulating the healthy cells to grow. See them growing until the area looks exactly like all the healthy tissue around it. With the third small hand have a jar of blue-golden salve made of sun and sky, which you rub over the healthy area in order to protect it. (If this has been a dry rash, then the jar should contain white palm oil that is rubbed over the area.) See, sense, and feel this healing taking place. When finished, raise your arms and hands toward the sun, seeing the rays telescope back into your palms, where the small hands and eyes are stored. Then breathe out and open your eyes.

SPINAL COLUMN PROBLEMS
(including lower-back problems)

Name: **Playing the Cord**
Intention: To heal the spinal column.
Frequency: Each morning, for 5 to 10 minutes, for a cycle
   of 21 days of use and 7 days off. If you want to continue,
   do two more cycles of 21 days with 7 days off in between.

The spinal column is the central pillar around which the physical body is organized. It is the body's main support structure, and as such it is subject to a great deal of mechanical stress—especially in our fast-moving, action-oriented society. Some prominent meanings I have found for spinal column problems are money woes and feelings of insecurity.

Continuous exertion may promote weakening of the spinal column. What subsequently may happen is that the vertebrae buckle, causing the gelatinous mass that acts as a pillow between the vertebrae to herniate. Buckling alone can cause pain and limitation of motion. Herniation can cause serious limitation of motion and severe pain. Another

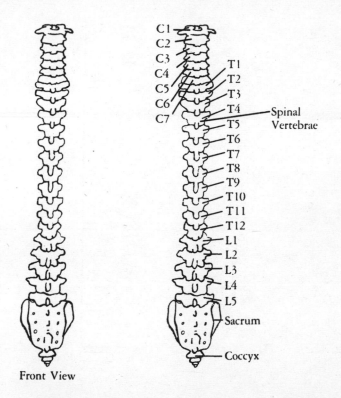

C1
C2
C3
C4
C5
C6
C7
T1
T2
T3
T4
T5
T6
T7
T8
T9
T10
T11
T12
L1
L2
L3
L4
L5
Sacrum
Coccyx
Spinal Vertebrae

Front View

problem is that calcium deposits may form at the tips of the vertebrae themselves. This buildup can create a narrowing of the space between the vertebrae, through which pass the nerves coming from the spinal column to different organs of the body. Pain and limitation of motion can result here as well. Sciatica is a common ailment resulting from such nerve pinching. The sciatic nerve runs from the spinal column through the buttocks, into the thigh, leg, foot, all the way down to the big toe.

The imagery exercise I advise for the spinal column is appropriate for all of the situations I have just described. It is the best one I have found for lower-back pain and lower-back problems in general. Before beginning the exercise, it

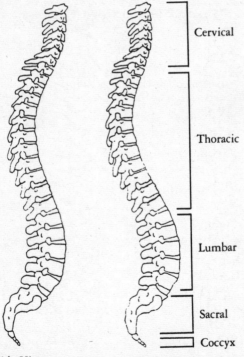

Cervical

Thoracic

Lumbar

Sacral

Coccyx

Side View

helps to familiarize yourself with the shape and number of vertebrae. There are seven cervical vertebrae, twelve thoracic or dorsal vertebrae; and five lumbar, sacral plate, and coccyx (in three segments) vertebrae.

Playing the Cord

Close your eyes, breathe out three times, and see your spinal column in front of you. If your pain or limitation is at the top of the column, start from below, and vice versa. For example, starting from above, see and touch C-1. See the color and hear the sound that it makes. If the color is anything other than white, use a brush, like one used to clean fingernails, and scrub the vertebra till it becomes gleaming white. If the sound you hear is not harmonious or in tune, manipulate the vertebra *very gently* between your thumb and forefinger until it is in place, or in alignment, and you hear a harmonious note. Then breathe out once and go to C-2. Repeat exactly the same procedure. Continue this, in sequence, throughout the spinal column. With reference to the coccyx, see the tilt of it. The normal coccyx tilts down and forward. If you see it at any other angle, it must be manipulated to the down and forward position until the harmonious note is heard. Remember to breathe out after working on each vertebra. After finishing this part, open your eyes. Then close your eyes again, breathe out three times, and start with the ligaments, tendons, and muscles alongside the coccyx, see yourself holding them with two hands and elongating and stretching them until they become glistening white. Then stretch the space between the coccyx and sacrum by placing one hand on each vertebra and gently spreading them apart. Clear away any filament around the space. Sense the blood flowing through the area of the muscles, tendons, and ligaments, and see light filling the space coming from above. When you are elongating and stretching, sense if there is movement in any part of your body and/or sensations in any organs. Continue in this same manner, stretching the space between the vertebrae in *ascending* order. That is, moving from sacrum -L-5, L5-L-4 L4-L-3, and so on, following the same directions as given above. The last stretching takes place between C-2 and C-1. After finishing at C-1, open your eyes. Then close your eyes and breathe out three times. Beginning at C-1, see and hear yourself playing your vertebrae like piano keys in descending order all the way through to the coccyx. Experience the feeling this gives. Then open your eyes.

STRESS

Name: **Stress Without Distress**
Intention: To remove distress.
Frequency: Daily as needed, for 30 seconds to 1 minute for
    each of the interrelated exercises.

Stress is the ordinary state of our everyday existence. It is with us almost always in our waking life (and sometimes while sleeping—for instance, when we are experiencing a nightmare); it is one of the essential features of living. Think about it: "I forgot my keys," "Oh, it's raining and I don't have an umbrella," "I've got a headache." On and on it goes. Stress or shocks are happening to us constantly. These shocks cannot be eliminated from our lives, nor should they be. They are awakeners that stimulate us to respond and to stay alert. Oftentimes we experience these shocks as painful. Our feeling then is called "distress." It is this distress, and not stress as such, that we have to contend with and manage. How we cope with distress shows our capacity for living a more or less balanced life. The following interrelated exercises are intended to help provide you with your own distress-management program. You should do the whole set of exercises.

Stress Without Distress

1. Close your eyes. Breathe out three times. See yourself feeding powerful giants. After finishing, open your eyes.

2. Close your eyes. Breathe out twice. See yourself making friends with hostile beings. Then open your eyes.

3. Close your eyes. Breathe out two times. See yourself knotting the head of a snake. After finishing, open your eyes.

4. Close your eyes. Breathe out three times. See yourself jumping on the back of a traveling dragon. After finishing, open your eyes.

5. Close your eyes. Breathe out once. See yourself calling forth the hidden inhabitants of a cavern. Then open your eyes.

6. Close your eyes. Breathe out twice. See yourself facing ghosts in an old castle. Then open your eyes.

7. Close your eyes. Breathe out three times. See yourself finding a powerful soul in a catacomb. Then open your eyes.

8. Close your eyes. Breathe out three times. See yourself leading a strange animal into a deep forest. Then open your eyes.

9. Close your eyes. Breathe out once. Look at a target that you have overshot. What is the proper action? Do you need a helper? Then open your eyes.

10. Close your eyes. Breathe out once. Look at a bird soaring upward when it is more opportune for the bird to remain low. What are you experiencing? Then open your eyes.

11. Close your eyes. Breathe out once. See how, in order to fulfill your true self, you have to struggle with the tide. Then open your eyes.

12. Close your eyes. Breathe out once. See why, after the struggle, we may then be still. Then open your eyes.

13. Close your eyes. Breathe out once. Know when it is good to speak and good to remain silent. Then open your eyes.

14. Close your eyes. Breathe out once. Know how, whatever is going on in our society, not to be impatient nor to surrender. Then open your eyes.

15. Close your eyes. Breathe out once. See that what is hastily made is quickly destroyed. Then open your eyes.

16. Close your eyes. Breathe out once. Looking into clear, quiet, calm water, see what you wish to see. After finishing, open your eyes.

17. Close your eyes. Breathe out once. Looking into clear, calm water, change your appearance as you would like to change it. After finishing, open your eyes.

SWELLING (known also as Edema. Also, see Premenstrual Syndrome)

Name: **Planting the Seeds**
Intention: To remove or relieve swelling.
Frequency: As needed until swelling is gone, for 2 to 3 minutes, every 1 to 2 hours.

Swelling of bodily tissues is known medically as "edema." This swelling can take place for various reasons: varicosities of veins, blockage of lymphatic drainage, trauma, or infection. Irrespective of the reason for the swelling, I recommend the following imagery exercise.

Planting the Seeds

Close your eyes. Breathe out three times and find yourself lying along a riverbank that has very fertile soil, like the bank of the Mississippi or the Nile. Encase the swollen area with this mud. Have with you quick-growing seeds, including those of the jade plant (a plant whose leaves swell to bursting with water absorbed from the soil) and plant them in the mud around your swelling. See, sense, and feel the seeds growing, the roots taking hold as they go down into your skin and into the swollen tissue. The roots draw up the fluid from your body—feel and sense the fluid being drawn and drained by the roots. See the seeds growing into plants that are bursting with fluid. See and know that your swelling is gone. Remove the mud cast from the area and plant the growth by the bank of the river. See the sun's rays coming down and drying off your formerly swollen area completely. Feel the warmth of the sun doing its work. Now see your body parts perfectly healthy. Breathe out and open your eyes.

THYROID DISTURBANCE

Name: **Red and Blue**
Intention: To make thyroid function normal.
Frequency: Four times a day (early morning, noon, twilight, bedtime), for 2 to 3 minutes, for three cycles of 21 days of use and 7 days off in between.

At that point go for a retest of the thyroid function. If it has improved, repeat the exercise program for another three cycles, this time twice a day—early morning and twilight. If there has been no change or even some worsening (not a bad sign), then repeat for three cycles, three times a day—early morning, twilight, and bedtime; and then another three cycles twice a day—early morning and bedtime. Sometimes your condition will get worse before it gets better, but within one to two weeks you should improve. If you do not improve after this time, see your doctor.

The thyroid gland is most important for helping to regulate the body's metabolism. This gland has the meaning of a

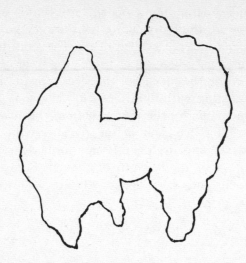

door, or shield, or forest. When there is thyroid trouble, I usually look for some issue regarding going through a door in life—that is, making a decision of moving from one phase of life to another. For example, one man I worked with was in the process of divorcing after a long marriage; he was making the transition painfully and had great reluctance in accepting the reality of the situation. He was "stepping through a new door," as he put it. He developed hyperthyroidism (overactive thyroid) in the course of this transition, as he moved toward being alone, unmarried, and in middle age. The suffering that results from this, and other similar transition situations, is kept in, or held on to, and is tucked into the thyroid. The thyroid then "speaks" about going through the door. Following is an imagery exercise to help you get through the door. It can be used for either overactive or underactive thyroid.

Red and Blue

Close your eyes. Breathe out three times. See yourself becoming very tall, with your arms becoming quite long, reaching your palms up to the sun. Take a piece of sun in your hands and place it in your thyroid (see diagram), seeing golden rays of light streaming to all parts of your body, giving health and well-being to your other glands. See red and blue channels of light crisscrossing in the thyroid, and know that your thyroid is functioning with normal hormone supply. See the pattern the crisscrossing makes, and see and sense a channel of red hormonal flow going from your pituitary to your thyroid, and a channel of blue flow going from your thyroid to your pituitary. When you see the flow of red and blue moving evenly and smoothly between pituitary and thyroid, know that your thyroid is functioning well. Then breathe out and open your eyes.

TUMORS (see Polyps and Tumors)

UPPER RESPIRATORY INFECTIONS

Name: **The Frightening Mask**
Intention: To clear up the infection.
Frequency: As needed until the infection is gone, three
    times every hour, every 2 to 3 hours, for 1 to 2 minutes.

Name: **Sounds of the Sinuses**
Intention: To clean and clear the sinuses.
Frequency: 1 to 2 minutes, every 30 minutes, until the
    sinuses are clear.

Upper respiratory infections most commonly involve the sinuses, nose, and throat; they less frequently affect the eustachian tubes of the ears and the upper part of the respiratory tree. Upper respiratory attacks are variously called flu or colds and sometimes laryngitis, bronchitis, or sinus-itis. But there is one thing that I have found associated with upper respiratory infections in general—and that is grief! The person with a cold or a flu is also crying over some thing or someone lost, or is responding to the memory of someone or something lost, or experiencing a transition in life. Separation and loss are the main ingredients for sad-ness, grief, crying, and upper respiratory disturbance. Put-ting your finger on the loss and acknowledging it openly to yourself can be beneficial in curtailing the symptoms.

It is not by chance that one of the most "contagious" times of the year for colds is the period between Thanksgiving and Christmas, on into the middle of January. This is the season when people are remembering what they once had and lost, or what they never had but wanted. We feel sad about families that once were but are no longer, or about families we wished we had but that didn't materialize in our lives. We see celebrations going on all around us, but we aren't part of them. The holiday season internally brings tearful reminders of emptiness and mourning and externally brings colds. The internal factor accounts in great measure for the stubborn resistance of this ailment against ordinary medical treatment.

Sinus trouble has the same meaning as upper respiratory infection in general. The eight sinuses are air chambers in the face. They ordinarily remain free of material, except when there is an infection in the area, and then they fill with fluid or pus. When this happens, the sinuses swell and you feel pain. Often there has been a "sinus," meaning a gap or separation, or the threat of a serious separation at the time of the infection. Each of the following exercises can be used for both sinusitis and colds.

The common cold is the bane of everyone's existence. We are always told that there is no cure for the common cold, that we just have to put up with it. At the beginning of chapter 1, I described **The River of Life,** which will pro-vide relief. **The Frightening Mask,** described below, should also help.

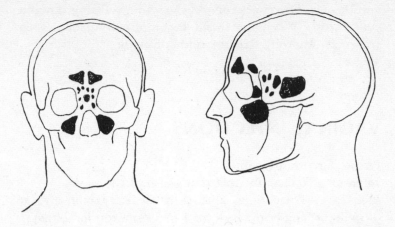

As you might know, antibiotics should be avoided in most of these situations, *especially* when there is absence of a high fever (101 degrees or more). Antibiotics should only be used when the presence of a bacterial infection has been confirmed by a nasal, sputum, or throat culture. You can certainly use either **The Frightening Mask** or **Sounds of the Sinuses** with some natural remedy such as saltwater nose drops, a gargle of epsom salts and warm water or a nasal wash of distilled water, 6–8 ounces, with one-quarter teaspoon of fine grained sea salt.

The Frightening Mask

Close your eyes and breathe out three times. Find a room of frightening masks. Select a mask and put it on. See, sense, and feel the departure of the cold demon. See him recoil. Then open your eyes.

Sounds of the Sinuses

Place your middle fingers or thumbs against the bridge of your nose. Close your eyes, breathe out three times, and hear the sound of the pain or clogging in your nose or sinuses.

Breathe out three times and feel the sound coursing through your throat. When the sound becomes harmonious, open your eyes, knowing that the cold is leaving.

VAGINAL INFECTIONS

Name: **Egyptian Healing**
Intention: To clear the infection and heal the vagina.
Frequency: Three times a day, in the early morning, at twilight, and before bed, for 1 to 3 minutes, for 21 days.

There are various sorts of vaginal infections connected with bacteria, viruses, or yeast. Infection can also stem from masturbatory or other mechanical irritations. Regardless of the type of infection, we are well served by trying to discover what emotional and social issues are feeding into the disturbance. These issues usually are inhibitions about or excesses of sexual activity. In any case, the infection reflects an imbalance and disharmony in sexuality. Following is an imagery exercise that can help bring you into balance. For this exercise it is useful to know that vagina is connected to vanilla, itself a form of orchid.

Egyptian Healing

Close your eyes and breathe out three times. Using the **Egyptian Healing** exercise (p. 45), see yourself entering the vanilla orchid. Smell the vital fragrance of vanilla. With one small hand take vanilla beans with you. Leave the orchid and enter your vagina, using your five eyes to see your way clearly. Survey the vaginal walls and in another small hand have a small golden brush with which you clean away all the infected cells thoroughly so that you see none left (remember that you are looking carefully at what you are doing all the time with

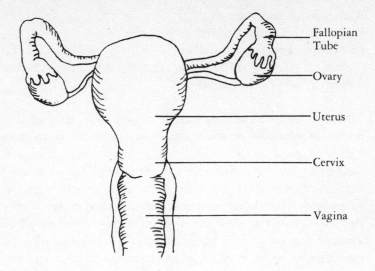

your five eyes). With your small hand containing the vanilla beans, plant the beans in the areas where you have removed the cells, and with your five eyes see beautiful white orchids growing out from the vaginal walls. With your third small hand have a golden watering can filled with pure rainwater, with which you water the orchids, watching the petals unfolding, smelling the aromatic fragrance of vanilla, and knowing that the vagina is healing perfectly. Leave the vagina and exit from your body by the way you entered. Then finish the **Egyptian Healing** exercise in the usual manner, and open your eyes.

WARTS

Name: **Egyptian Healing**
Intention: To remove warts.
Frequency: Three times a day, for 2 to 3 minutes, for 21 days. If more is needed, use for two more 21-day cycles, with 7 days off in between.

Name: **Reverse Face**

Intention: To remove warts; to heal the skin.

Frequency: Four times a day, for 1 to 3 minutes, for 21 days. If more is needed, use for two more 21-day cycles with 7 days off in between.

These pushy little critters appear on the skin, are usually brown or blackish brown in color, seem to be connected with the presence of a virus, and, while not especially dangerous, can be cosmetically unappealing. They are usually cut or burned off, but tend to recur, hence the need for an imagery exercise to get rid of them permanently. When they emerge on the face, warts are to be considered a sign of some physical or emotional imbalance. This should prompt you to look further regarding an emotional conflict and see your doctor about any physical issue.

To treat warts on the face with imagery, I often use a combination of two exercises—**Egyptian Healing,** described on p. 45, followed by **Reverse Face.** I recommend that patients continue these exercises—a cycle of **Egyptian Healing** (21 days of use, 7 days off) followed by **Reverse Face** (21 days of use, 7 days off), until the warts have cleared up. For warts elsewhere, **Egyptian Healing** used alone will suffice.

Egyptian Healing

Following the directions for **Egyptian Healing** (p. 45) turn your five eyes to examine your wart(s) carefully. Then in one small hand have a ball of fine golden thread and with it tie a knot at the base of the wart(s). In another small hand have a tube that emits a beam of white laser light. Shine this light directly on the wart(s), seeing it (them) shrivel up and fall off. In your third small hand use a soft golden brush to wipe away the debris that's left, and see the first pink skin underneath. In your fourth small hand have a golden mirror. Look at your healing skin reflected there, looking like the healthy skin around it. Then follow the procedure for ending the Egyptian Healing exercise as described on p. 45. Afterwards, open your eyes.

Reverse Face

Close your eyes. Breathe out three times, and find yourself at a cool, crystal-clear, fresh-flowing mountain stream (or any healing body of water). See your face there (or the part with the warts) and then remove it, turn it inside out, and wash it thoroughly in the stream. See all the waste products as black or gray strands being carried away in the fast-flowing stream with its spiral currents. After your face (or other body part) is thoroughly washed, hang it out to dry in the sun. See it healing from the inside, looking like all the other healthy tissue around it. Then turn the face right side out and put it back in place, seeing that the warts have disappeared. Then open your eyes.

WORRY

Names: **Removing the Yoke** and **Lightening the Burdens**
Intention: To relieve worry.
Frequency: Anytime you feel worried; 30 seconds to 1
   minute for **Removing the Yoke,** 1 to 2 minutes for
   Lightening the Burden.

Like all disturbing emotions, worry involves time frames over which we have no control. These time frames represent either the past, which we can't change, or the future, which is impossible for us to determine. Most of us mistakenly believe that the personal past and personal future are more important than the present moment. However, the present is where happiness resides. Most of us say that we want to be happy and that we keep searching for happiness. This search takes us into many blind alleys. The three major ones are the past, the future, and living *for,* not in, the present (the former otherwise known as hedonism). The "happiness" to which I refer means living *in* the moment. To get to this moment, remove or ease the yoke that is now choking you. *Worry,* remember, means "to be strangled." If you can see yourself easing up, you have made an inroad into your worry. Anytime you feel choked with worry, wear your yoke more easily, with the intention of eliminating worry.

Removing the Yoke

Close your eyes. Breathe out once, and see whatever it is that is strangling you, and either ease it, loosen it, or remove it from around your neck. Notice then how your breathing improves, and at the same time know that your worry has evaporated. Then open your eyes.

Lightening the Burdens

Close your eyes, breathe out once, and see yourself removing your burdens, burning them, burying the ashes, and sensing how light your body becomes. Notice how your breathing deepens as the body becomes lighter, knowing that your worry has been removed. Then open your eyes.

CHAPTER FIVE

Exercises for Health

In this chapter are several exercises to help you maintain or heighten your general health and well-being. They are not aimed at specific maladies but rather at the processes by which we can all become more of what we are meant to be.

A BODYMIND CHECKUP

Name: **The Lake of Health and The Field of Health**
Intention: To see your state of health.
Frequency: As needed, once for up to 3 minutes.

If, besides visiting your doctor, you want to do some periodic checking on the state of your health, following are two imagery exercises you can count on to provide information. The axiom that holds true in the world of imagery is that the image doesn't lie. Becoming receptive to this truth can be immensely helpful in developing trust in yourself, and it will be especially beneficial in assessing your state of affairs.

A related imagery event that can reveal some oncoming trouble is your night dreams. Here you should pay attention to the appearance of individual, bright colors. A striking blue, red, green, orange, or yellow can bespeak some thyroid, vascular, gallbladder, liver, or kidney trouble, respectively. I would suggest that you go for a checkup when this happens. The one exception that I have found is the appearance of red in a night dream during menstruation. This is a normal accompaniment in dream life to the biological event of a woman's period.

The Lake of Health

Close your eyes. Breathe out three times and see yourself high up in the Andes at a lake that is at eighteen thousand feet. Tell the lake that you want to know the state of your health and that you want it to reveal your outer and inner body to you. Then look into the crystal-clear, quiet water and see yourself inside and out. (If you are healthy, you will characteristically see a golden color, pure pink, blue, or green. If you are ill, a gray, black, or bluish pink will appear at the site of the disturbance.) Then open your eyes.

The Field of Health

Close your eyes. Breathe out three times and see yourself as a general outside your tent at the head of the field of your body. Your bugler is next to you. You have a large golden flag blowing in the breeze at the top of your tent. At all important points on the field of your body are other tents with flags flying and buglers stationed next to them. Have your bugler blow his bugle and hear each bugler at each tent answer in turn. See the flags blowing at the same time and see their colors. Then open your eyes. If any sound is discordant, or a flag does not blow or shows a black or gray color, some change is taking place that bespeaks some disturbance or illness. It would be advisable then to consult your doctor.

BURYING THE PAST
(see also **Cleansing** and **Retracing the Past**)

Name: **Burying the Past**
Intention: To remove the influence of the past.
Frequency: Once a week, for 3 to 5 minutes, for three
    weeks.

Many people find that they cannot let go of the past. They may feel haunted by it, regret it, feel trapped by it, feel guilty about it, and so on. The intrusion of the past prevents us from being able to function productively. Harping on it can't change it; we seem only to keep experiencing more pain. The following exercise, aptly called **Burying the Past,** may help to relieve some of that tension and help to put the past to rest.

Burying the Past

Close your eyes. Breathe out three times. You are walking along a country path. The path is cluttered with rocks, which you clear in order to make it passable. At the end of the path you find a tree. Sit by the tree; from the ground, pick up a leaf and on it write all that has pained you from your past, all the regrets and all the obstacles from the past that inhibit you from going forward. Use the sap on the leaf as ink with which to write. Then dig a hole, knowing that you are going to bury the leaf and that the past, although buried, is still alive but will eventually disintegrate. Indicate when you want the past to disintegrate by writing a date on the leaf, then place the leaf in the hole, bury it with dirt, and quickly go back to where you started, seeing if there is anything different on the path. Then open your eyes.

CLEANSING

Name: **The Garden of Eden**
Intention: To prepare yourself for everyday life in a positive way.
Frequency: Daily, in the early morning, for up to 3 minutes.

This cleansing exercise is a wonderful way to start the day. It puts you in a good mood, and it also raises the level of your immune system. I often ask my patients to clean physically as well; clean out the clutter from their homes or an area in their homes on a regular basis, with the intention that they are cleaning themselves out internally at the same time.

The Garden of Eden

Close your eyes. Breathe out three times, and imagine yourself leaving your home and going out into the street (those of you who can descend a staircase should do so). Leave the street and see yourself descending into a valley, meadow, or garden, and go to the center of it. Find there a golden feather duster, whisk broom, or hand rake (depending on your preference, or the degree of cleansing you need). With this tool, quickly clean yourself thoroughly from top to bottom, including your extremities. See how you look and feel, knowing that you have cleaned away all the dead cells from the outside of your body and all the gloom and confusion from the inside.

Put down the tool and hear from your right the sound of a flowing stream or brook. Go there and kneel by its edge. Take the fresh-flowing, crystal-clear, cool water in your cupped hands and splash it over your face, knowing that you are washing away all the impurities from the outside of your body. Then take the fresh-flowing, crystal-clear, cool water in your cupped hands and drink it very slowly, knowing that you are washing away all the impurities from the inside of your body. Feel and sense yourself refreshed, tingling, energized, and more awake.

Get up from the stream and find a tree at the edge of the meadow. Sit under the tree that has branches hanging down with green leaves. Then with your back against the trunk, take in the pure oxygen that the leaves emit, together with the oxygen in the form of a blue-golden light from the sun and the sky that comes between the leaves. Breathe out carbon dioxide in the form of gray smoke, which the leaves take up and convert into oxygen. This oxygen is given off by the leaves and comes through the trunk, entering your body through your pores. You are thus making a cycle of breathing with the tree and are breathing as one with the tree. Let your fingers and toes curl into the earth, like roots, and draw up its energy. Stay there for a long moment, taking in what you need. Then get up from the tree and see how you look and feel.

Keep the image and feelings for yourself as you leave the garden and return to your street. Go back to your home by the way you went, and return to your chair. Then breathe out and open your eyes.

GENERAL WELL-BEING

Name: **The Red Suit**
Intention: To maintain general health.
Frequency: Once a day, for 2 minutes, every day.

A simple way to produce physiological changes through imagery is imaginal jogging, a natural accompaniment to a physical exercise program that can improve its effectiveness. Even for those of you who don't exercise, or who find it boring, imaginal jogging can be beneficial. Recently a study was done at a Canadian hospital where patients undergoing rehabilitation from heart attack were divided into two groups. One group was given a typical physical exercise program; the other group was asked to perform the same program imaginally rather than physically. When the recovery rates of the two groups were compared, the imagery group was found to have recovered much more quickly.

The Red Suit

Close your eyes. Breathe out three times and see yourself putting on a red jogging suit and red sneakers. See yourself going out of your home or apartment and walking to the park. Enter the park and begin to run around it clockwise, becoming aware of everything you see. Become aware of what you sense and feel, of the wind passing by you. Become aware of your stride and your breathing. Notice the trees, grass, and sky. Complete the run by coming back to the point at which you started. Walk out of the park and back to your home. Take off the jogging clothes, shower, dry off, and see yourself put on the clothes you are going to wear for that day. Then open your eyes.

GIVING YOURSELF A NEW START

Name: **Egyptian Rebirth**
Intention: To give yourself a new start, a hopeful look to the future, a sense of purpose and meaning.
Frequency: Once, for 5 to 10 minutes. This exercise is done only once every two years.

This is a general healing exercise—healing in the sense of becoming whole—that will help you give yourself a new sense of purpose. Sometimes life can become routine or dull, or we are no longer inspired or satisfied by what we are doing. This exercise will enable you to shape new possibilities for yourself.

Egyptian Rebirth

Close your eyes. Breathe out once and see yourself as a scarab beetle deep in the earth at the base of a root, drawing nourishment from it. Gather seeds from the surrounding earth. Take part of the root and make a ball, using saliva and earth to keep the ball together. Begin pushing the ball with your front legs upward and ahead like this

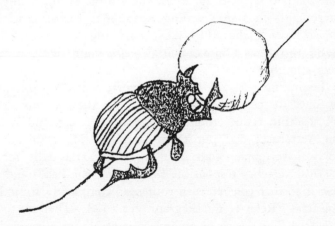

—until you reach the earth's surface. Find a soft spot and, tucking the ball against your abdomen, use your forelegs to make a hole in the crust, and come out onto the surface. Stay there a few moments, breathing now as an external creature and no longer an internal one. Feel the chest and lungs expanding and see the carapace (the hard shell equivalent to your back) looking straight and long as you stand up in your clear green casing. Next, feel the soft inside of your scarab body moving in a supple way within the rigid frame of the long backbone, which is seen as bright and straight. Then, using your faceted eyes, which can turn to look in all directions, see a river directly behind you and a mountain in front of you.

You have to climb the mountain and to push the ball in front of you, using your forelegs, shoulders, and lower back. The ball now has grass adhering to it, making it larger and larger in front of you, until you can no longer see where you are going. The ball is also getting heavier and heavier while you are climbing. Make sure that you don't lose the ball; otherwise, you will have to retrieve it and start over again. When you arrive at the top of the mountain, see, in the distance, the target or goal that you want. Then roll the ball down or off the mountaintop, seeing it hit the target squarely and exploding, sending all the seeds scattering, knowing that they must land and take root. Then stand upright as a human being, seeing your back becoming very straight.

Beginning with the lowest vertebra, touch each one, one by one, to see if they are in place. If they are not, clear off the thin tissue around the vertebrae, clean and stretch the vertebrae, and put them in place. Move up to the cervical vertebrae, coming now to the atlas (the second cervical vertebra responsible for turning the head) and adjust it so that you can turn your head completely around on the atlas. (Refer to the diagram on p. 173.) Then go to the axis (the first cervical vertebra, responsible for allowing the head to bend forward and backward), and adjust it so that you can bend your head completely forward so that your chin touches your breastbone. Afterward, you find yourself becoming, or have already become, very tall.

Your head is perfectly straight and your double chin (if you have one) has become flat. Feel every joint and articulation moving freely, beginning with the toes, to the bones of the foot, to the ankle, to the knee, to the tendons stretching behind the knee, to the pelvis and hip bones, feeling them rotate. Feel the tendons stretching along your spinal column. Now stretch all the way up to the sun and take some of it in your hands. When elongating to take the sun, feel your hands and arms stretching, knowing that your hands are your antennae. With the sun, burn off the fat from your abdomen (if you have any) and massage your back. Then burn off the fat from your double chin (if such exists). Warm the rest of your body with it. Place it in your solar plexus (about one inch below the lower end of your breastbone), giving heat to it, and the solar plexus sends this heat to the rest of the body. Wash your hands in the sun, and afterward throw it back in place.

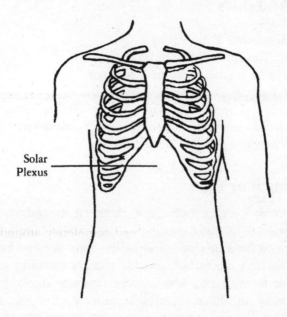

Solar Plexus

Then look at the place of your goal and see how the trees and all other vegetation have grown there, knowing that all has come to fruition there, and see it bright. Run down the mountain lightly to the bottom, run to the river, and jump across into a bright, large, clear, open space and enjoy being there. Go now to the river and bathe in it, knowing that all is repaired. Bathe for a short time. Come out and sit under a tree to rest. Then *physically* open your eyes and see the river, space, mountain, and trees, with flowers and fruits. See your eyes without sadness and in a new way. Know that what you want to accomplish will be finished in two years.

RELAXATION

Name: **Becoming Blue Light**
Intention: To achieve inner relaxation.
Frequency: As needed for 1 to 3 minutes.

This exercise is for the occasions when the breathing-out exercise is not enough to produce inner relaxation, or in general when you feel you need to relax.

Becoming Blue Light

Close your eyes. Breathe out three times and see the oxygen you are inhaling coming in the form of blue-golden light formed by a mixture of cloudless blue sky and bright golden sun and the carbon dioxide you are exhaling going out in the form of gray smoke, like cigarette smoke being carried away in the air and disappearing. See the light become blue light as it enters your body, comes out of your heart, and travels evenly, gently, and smoothly through the arteries and capillaries, knowing that as it does you are becoming relaxed. When it has traveled throughout your entire body, open your eyes.

RETRACING THE PAST

Name: **Retracing the Past, Parts 1 & 2**
Intention: To remove the influence of your past.
Frequency: Once a day, for 7 minutes for each part, for 21
  days.

This imagery exercise provides a powerful way to wash out
past influences and past traumas in your life. It is done in
two parts. The first corrects the influence of the external
world on you from earliest life until now, recognized as
events and places. The second corrects your own internal
influences on your life from earliest childhood until now,
recognized as faults and errors. It is quite successful in
helping you to wipe out persistent negative beliefs and
experiences.

By correcting events, places, faults, and errors, I mean
that you correct either your attitude or your beliefs regarding the experience, or you correct the experience itself. You
can look at past events as beliefs that you have held on to in
your memory. Through this exercise, you can remove the
effects of these events by shifting your attitude or beliefs
about them or by washing them away. You then create for
yourself new beliefs by living the corrected events with a
different past and a new present. Once the new beliefs are
set in place, they will be expressed as new experiences in
your life!

Retracing the Past, Parts 1 & 2

Close your eyes and breathe out three times. Looking into
a mirror, see, sense, feel, know, and live in chronological
order all the *significant* disturbing places or events of your
life that you can recall from earliest childhood or infancy
until the present moment. After completing that, keep your
eyes closed. Breathe out once, and looking into the mirror

see, sense, feel, know, and live yourself correcting these disturbing events and places in *reverse* chronological order, starting with the present moment and going back to earliest childhood or infancy. For events and/or places incapable of being corrected, see yourself washing them out of the left side of the mirror using a fireman's hose. Keep your eyes closed. Breathe out once and, looking into the mirror, see, sense, feel, know, and live again these now-corrected events and places with a different past and a new now, seeing how you have to become in one year from now, two years from now, and five years from now. When you are finished, open your eyes.

Afterward, go through *exactly the same procedure* for part 2. This time, instead of considering disturbing events and places, the instruction is to see, sense, feel, know, and live the significant faults and errors of your life. After completing this part, open your eyes.

SELF-RENEWAL

Name: **Rejuvenation**
Intention: To revive you, give you a sense of renewed purpose.
Frequency: Once a week for three weeks, 30 seconds to 1
    minute for each exercise.

When you're feeling uneasy and need a tonic to revive you, or if you need rejuvenating or a sense of renewed purpose, try the following exercises.

Rejuvenation

1. Close your eyes. Breathe out once. Use a spade to dig up emotions in order to find something hidden. Take what you find for yourself. Then open your eyes.

2. Close your eyes. Breathe out once. Defuse a live bomb. Then open your eyes.

3. Close your eyes. Breathe out once. See an animal coming toward you on an incline. Then open your eyes.

4. Close your eyes. Breathe out once. Herd wild horses into a corral. Then open your eyes.

5. Close your eyes. Breathe out once. Be someone being someone else. Then open your eyes.

6. Close your eyes. Breathe out once. You are wrapped in bandages up to the neck. How do you feel? Unwrap the bandages and make them into a ball. Then open your eyes.

7. Close your eyes. Breathe out once. Make your way walking backward into a panther or leopard skin. See and sense what happens. Then open your eyes.

CHAPTER SIX

Eight Pointers for Developing Your Own Imagery

Once you begin working with imagery, you quickly become comfortable with it and you begin using images that belong to you. Up to this point, I have provided you with exercise blueprints. Now, to help you devise your own exercises, I will give you eight pointers to assist you in making imagery your own tool.

1. The first pointer is that you always start with your point of trouble. Whatever the immediate problem is, physical or mental, you face it.

One of my patients so suffered from panic and fear of the dark that staying awake with the light on seemed to him the only remedy. Following is the exercise I recommended. The intention, of course, is to sleep peacefully.

Sunset Exercise

At bedtime, turn on all the lights in the bedroom, sit upright in a chair with your eyes closed, breathe out three times, and see yourself in the middle of a meadow. It is pitch dark, but you know that the sun is about to come up. You see the darkness disappearing and dawn breaking and it becomes a bright, sunny day. Suddenly, you become aware of a light sunshower, washing over you from head to foot, quieting and soothing you as it falls. Then the sunshower stops, and you imagine yourself lying in the meadow, laying your head on a velvety tuft of grass. Look at the clear blue sky. See the sun high in the sky, then beginning to set. Watch it set till it sinks below the horizon, knowing that as it does, you are able to go to sleep. After finishing, open your eyes, turn off the lights, and go to bed.

As you can see, I start this exercise with exposure to the immediate fear—in this case, of the dark. Also in imagery work, we always start with the reality of what the person is experiencing—in this case, the reality of insomnia.

For a person who is afraid of flying, I recommend the following exercise.

Flying Free

Close your eyes. Breathe out three times. Calm and quiet yourself, and see yourself in a meadow. Sit there and sense a soft breeze blowing over you. Hear the birds chirping. See a cloudless sky and the sun above you. After quieting yourself, see yourself boarding an airplane, wearing a protective device of your own choice. Take off in the plane and make the entire flight dressed in your protective gear, knowing that nothing can hurt you. See, sense, and feel your now-invulnerable self; sitting as either the pilot or copilot, direct the plane. Note your emotions and sensations as you go. Then land safely, alight from the plane, touch the ground, and remove your protection. Breathe out slowly once, keeping for yourself all that has been positive on the flight. Then open your eyes.

*   *   *

Again we start with the point of trouble—the immediate problem. This approach applies to any ailment, even one as severe as cancer. I asked one of my patients to visualize her cancer. She saw two monsters coming out of a cave. I suggested she use any weapon she needed to protect herself and fight off the monsters.

Another way of starting with the trouble—say, an earache—is simply to enter your body at the point of pain and see whatever image comes to you. Then do what you need to do to heal your wound.

2. The second pointer is that *any image you find is correct for you.* Do not make any judgments about the kind of images that come, as to whether they make sense or are worth-while, and do not try to interpret them or figure out their meaning.

You will often find useful imagery coming to you from the way you speak of your problems or from your night dreams. Paying attention to these areas can yield many sorts of images to use. For instance, a depressed woman, describing her mood, said, "I feel like I am at the bottom of a well." In the word-image "well," she provided an image to use in helping herself *out* of her mood.

3. The third pointer is that you should *trust that you will be able to make use of your image.* For instance, if you were like the woman who felt she was at the bottom of a well, you would want to find your way out of the well by climbing up and out using a ladder you may find there, knowing that as you ascend, your mood is lifting. Remember that anything can happen in imagination, which makes finding the ladder there rather easy. You can bring with yourself the necessary means to benefit you in imagery activity.

4. The fourth pointer concerns the effect that disturbances have on our body rhythms. When we are sick, our body rhythms become too fast or too slow. For example, a malfunctioning thyroid can be either underactive or overactive. With an underactive thyroid, we become too heavy and/or too sleepy; with an overactive thyroid, too thin and

prone to insomnia. Cancer offers another example: there is a quickening of the rhythm of the affected organ, and its cells are multiplying with incredible rapidity.

In using imagery you need to be concerned with the rhythms of your disturbance. The general rule is to *use the opposite of what you have*. If you are suffering from a "too fast" condition such as: stress, rapid heartbeat, or anxiety, use quieting imagery to slow down the system. If your problem is a "too slow" condition such as: fatigue, some types of depression, or gall or kidney stones, use fast images. How will you know if your condition is too fast or too slow? You need only turn your attention to your ailment for a minute. You will feel the rhythm of your body and know whether it is fast or slow. You can also discuss this with your doctor.

Consider the woman at the bottom of the well. She was depressed (a slow condition) and needed to climb up, which should be quick. On the other hand, if you have a fast heartbeat, you could imagine your heart as an outboard motorboat moving along on a sunny day. Then you could shut the motor off—giving yourself the opposite of what you have—and see and sense the boat drifting on a windless waterway, knowing that the heart is slowing down.

5. The fifth pointer for using imagery is that *you can apply a paradoxical approach to the problem you are working with.*

This point is not as immediately clear as the others, I know. A paradoxical approach means to apply what apparently makes the least sense in a given situation, something that does not obey your logical approach to things. For instance, when you are feeling pain, you understandably want to turn and retreat from it. The paradox here is to do exactly the opposite. Join the pain, become the pain, shake hands with the pain. This seemingly nonsensical step can give you control over the pain because the act of merging with it—without labeling it with terms such as "awful," "terrible," "horrible"—can render it almost powerless.

This is so, I believe, because all modes of experiencing

sensation, emotion, images, or words, are *thought forms*. Whatever way you process your experience, you are in the midst of a form. When you recognize your pain, for example, you are actually entering into a thought form. Some of you may see pain as an image; some of you may sense or feel it without an accompanying image. It always assumes a shape when you enter it. This is true for *all* experiences, whether they are inner and subjective or external and objective. When you enter a thought form, you will find a transformation taking place in which either a new creative form will emerge (an image, a feeling, or a sensation) or the disturbing form will disappear. And with either of these responses, you will find relief.

In short, when we are confronted by something disturbing or fearful, we characteristically turn away. The paradox is to confront that which is distressing—*turn to it, not away from it*. Do with it what before you would never have dreamt of doing—go *toward* it. Greet it! Welcome it! Join it!

6. The sixth pointer concerns the inner guides that sometimes appear when you do imagery. None of the exercises in this book requires an inner guide, and you can achieve great success and wonderful results without ever meeting a guide. Nonetheless, if you should encounter an inner guide during the course of your imagery, *do not hesitate, under any circumstances, to use it to serve you*.

You may have read or heard about inner guides. They have a long and remarkable history in the Western spiritual tradition, in which they appear as angels. Angels are referred to throughout the Old and New Testaments and in the Koran. Angelology (the study of angels) is found in Judaism, Christianity, and Islam. All three traditions mention that everyone is born with a guardian angel who can be summoned simply by asking for it.

Inner guides/guardian angels come to you in the form in which you are prepared or able to receive them. They can appear as animals, humans, otherworldly creatures, or whatever other way your perception will allow. At the outset of trying to help yourself, you can call on the inner guide/guardian angel to help you. The calling can be done silently and inwardly. They will not come if not asked.

This pointer has a corollary: *If you doubt the reality of the inner guides/guardian angels, it is unlikely that you will be able to call on them.* Your skepticism will interfere with your ability to summon them. But if you are willing to suspend your skepticism and try, you may be surprised by the results.

7. The seventh pointer concerns the relationship between imaginal reality and everyday reality. The key is this: *Whatever you discover for yourself, whatever answer you may find, whatever instruction you receive, to gain its benefits you need to carry it out in your everyday reality as a lived experience.* You need to manifest the inner belief as an outer experience. For example, one patient discovered a room in which a table was laden with all sorts of beautiful vegetables and fruits. He "realized" from this experience that he had to change his diet. He became a vegetarian, much to the benefit of his health.

Another patient discovered an amethyst in her imagery. She subsequently bought one and wore it around her neck. She found that her tendency to drink too much alcohol diminished markedly. She then discovered that the amethyst had been known in medical lore as a gemstone to be worn to curb alcohol intake.

What you find in your imagery work are pictorial instructions that reveal to you what you need. Your inner, knowing being is there, ready to serve you. Use him/her/it freely, with his/her/its blessing.

8. A final, essential pointer: *Above all, do not compare yourself to anyone else.* It is not important that you get better faster or quicker than someone else who has a similar problem. Your only focus should be you, establishing your own health.

*   *   *

Some people worry that imagery is a form of self-absorption, misunderstanding it as an indulgence in our own habitual fantasies. An individual's health is deeply involved in healthy human relationships; and imagery work, far from inducing self-absorption, reveals the importance of relationships and shows you how to maintain them without sacrificing yourself to them or to the purposes or manipulations of other people.

Further, once you begin imagery work, you begin immediately to take care of yourself.

All this has been summed up in the wise formula of Rabbi Hillel, who lived in the first century:

> If I am not for me, who will be for me?
> If I am only for myself, what am I?
> If not now, when?

CHAPTER SEVEN

The Positive Beliefs of Healing Imagery

Imagery work can help us all to be healthier. It can also bring us a deeper, more meaningful life. In this closing chapter, I want to talk about the rich import of imagery.

A friend of mine was changing a light bulb. As he was removing the old one, he found that it did not turn easily. He applied more pressure, so much so that the glass broke, severely cutting his hand. He rushed to the hospital emergency room, where he required four stitches to close the wound. In the course of his examination, his blood pressure was found to be elevated. He realized that something had to be done to control this pressure. This something involved his losing 30 pounds and changing his diet.

I tell this story to illustrate two important factors regarding the process of health. The first is that what seems at first "bad" may turn out to have some "good" results. My friend's "bad" cut on his hand had a "good" result—his discovery of the high blood pressure, which he then brought under control.

The second factor is that for many of us, illness alerts us to a need to make some correction in our lives. In a way, illness may be a gift. Personally, I believe this gift is a spiritual one, coming as an act of love from God in which we may have to suffer a bit to get the message.

Often it is suffering that eventually makes us start to take steps to effect change in our lives. Many people do not heed the message of suffering and experience pain persistently. Others seek relief from the suffering without learning anything from the experience. Some seek relief at any cost and either become addicted to drugs or fall prey to dubious or unscrupulous healing practices, whether performed by someone with medical training or not. I believe that the viewpoint that suffering is "bad" itself perpetuates suffering—the very thing we are trying to overcome. This viewpoint stops us from looking further into the matter.

You might say, "Okay, what happened has been sent to teach me something. But I'm confused because I can't figure out what I'm supposed to learn, and I'm no better off than before." I could not disagree more. The realization that nothing is wholly bad is a significant first step along the path of self-awareness. Once we establish the habit of realizing that we are blessed by being given challenges, our lives are that much more enriched. My experience as a clinician clearly establishes that when this shift in attitude takes place, answers come to us, rather spontaneously, about the meaning of an illness and its place in our lives.

My essential point here is that we create the situation of suffering in which we find ourselves. When something "goes bad," that is the signal that we have forgotten this fact, we have forgotten ourselves. The next step is to remember ourselves and to start looking at our beliefs, which we have created.

When negative beliefs come to you, often in the form of negative thoughts and emotions, accept them as a gift and be thankful for their appearance. *Know* that even a negative belief can be a positive force in your life. It is an expression of life force. It is, in fact, keeping you in life. It is a channel to freedom—freedom from being enslaved by negative thoughts and feelings, and freedom to create a whole and happy life. The negative belief is a reminder to us to use our will and our reason to put ourselves back on course. It is always a signal to us that we have forgotten ourselves and that we need to return to our center.

The old saying goes, "Seek and you shall find." It is true. The rest of the adage is equally true: "Ask and you will be answered. Knock and the door will be opened to you." First, acknowledge the gift of beliefs; second, ask what you can do with this gift; third, know that what you learn, you can apply it to your life.

Do *not* ask why something that seems negative has happened to you. The more you ask this question, the more you will suffer and the more handcuffed you will feel. You will end up burdening yourself with more beliefs to wade through. Accept what has happened as facts of your personal history. You *can* change how you respond to intrusions of the past into your present life. You can always alter your *relationship* to what has happened by creating a new belief. Imagery can help you see events in a new way—for example, through an exercise such as **Retracing the Past,** in chapter 5. If you have already tried this exercise, you may have found that the imagery gave you a sense of hope and provided a new option for reacting to a past conditioning.

I believe that the techniques of imagery and the use of imagination have come along at this point in history as reflections of the needs of contemporary people in contemporary life. The tenets and attitudes of modern life seem to have left many of us feeling disempowered and unable to cope with the stresses to which we are exposed. Particularly debilitating are what we can call "mass consciousness beliefs" of impending world disasters such as nuclear war, famine, and mass extinction. It is difficult to extricate ourselves from such beliefs, especially when we have contributed to them.

I see all this from my perspective as a physician and clinician working daily with people suffering from diseases such as cancer and AIDS. I have made investigations into these disease processes and have discovered, for example, that according to the latest statistics of the American Cancer Society, 985,000 new cases of cancer showed up in 1988, a huge number. There are large environmental factors at play here. Consider, for example, that the highly industrialized states have the highest incidence of cancer per capita in the country. I believe this connection is not coincidental. The ordinary stresses of making our way on this earth have been compounded by the stresses created by the assault on the planet, which has led to the contamination of earth, air, and water.

You and I together have created all of these environmental hazards. They stem from the mass belief that industrial production is necessary for us to live the "good life," that industrial production will provide us with the antidote to scarcity, which most of us think is the thief at the back door of our lives. It may, but at what price? Yet again, it may not be at all.

The immune system and the ozone layer are both defense systems, the former for us and the latter for our planet, and both today are under attack. The defenses of both the earth and its inhabitants are being besieged directly. Some have gone so far as to declare that AIDS is just the beginning of the invasion of the retroviruses. (Retroviruses attack the immune system directly—a phenomenon that has never happened before in recorded history.)

But we need not give in to prognostications of despair. I believe that the use of imagination is one among a group of processes that can bring about the self-awareness and self-remembrance that will empower and restore people to their natural state of self-autonomy. It is the basis for a new form of education.

The means for healing ourselves and our planet are here. Controlled use of the imagination is one of the most powerful and readily accessible of these means. What you can do for yourself and for our common life with a mind that is free—a mind that no one can take away from you, even if you were placed in physical captivity—is limitless.

In my office, I teach people how to use the tools I have described in this book. Our work tends to go quickly, and the cost-benefit ratio for the people who work with me is amazingly low. Once people have started becoming their own authority, they no longer need me, except for an occasional checkup. I can say with confidence that the therapeutic approach outlined here puts into our hands a tool that permits us to become our own authority and our own healer. When this happens, we can accord doctors their proper roles—as resources to aid us in our task of restoring our health.

It is clear to me that disease and negative emotional states are images of negative beliefs. The nature of disease seems to be physical, while the nature of emotional states seems to be mental. But both are images, which means that they are actually our own mental creations. If you can accept this, or at least consider it, you are on the way to becoming the author of yet a new chapter in your life.

Look around and you will find innumerable negative messages bombarding you—not to mention the constant stresses of misinformation flooding in from friends, family, and others of similar sincerity, seeking, with all good intention, to pronounce judgments, advise without benefit of experience, and act generally as your authority. Your beliefs are generating it! All of it is your creation! Knowing this puts you on the road to becoming your own authority.

People who take it upon themselves to make the effort to love themselves, devictimize themselves, and extend this perspective to the universe find that the universe responds. It is as simple as changing your beliefs.

In the ancient Judeo-Christian wisdom we are told that at each moment in our existence we are faced with choosing life or choosing death. Choosing life is what being alive is all about. When we choose life via positive beliefs, we align ourselves with the rhythms, harmony, abundance, and grace of the universe. Have absolutely no doubt about this. It is a promise that has been made to us from the beginning.

Imagery is a positive belief system. It enables us to choose life. If such an opportunity for healing and salvation has been offered, why not take advantage of it?

A great sage, who was a dear and close friend, gave me an incredible insight before her death. I had asked her to tell me the meaning of life. She said, "Become a law unto yourself." Because she had the gift for saying so much in so few words, I asked her if she could expand on that thought. She complied readily, and in her characteristically pithy manner she added: "Become your own authority." For me, the statement was a revelation and was all that needed to be said. For you, I would add: Let your personal trouble be the starting point for taking charge of your life. Use imagery to help yourself become your own authority. Let your beliefs create your experience and say *yes* to life.

About the Author

Gerald Epstein, M.D., is a physician who has been a pioneer in the uses of mental imagery. He is the author of many books and articles on imagery, including his groundbreaking book *Waking Dream Therapy: Dream Process As Imagination*. Dr. Epstein is an assistant clinical professor of psychiatry at Mt. Sinai Medical Center in New York City. He gained his formal training as a medical doctor at New York Medical College and took his psychiatric residency at Kings County Hospital (Brooklyn, N.Y.). He received over twenty-two years of training and apprenticeship in the functions of the mind. He completed training and practiced as a psychoanalyst before apprenticing for nine years as a student of imagery methods with Mme. Colette Aboulker Muscat in Jerusalem. For thirteen years, Dr. Epstein edited *Tne Journal of Psychiatry and Law,* which he co-founded. He has been in private practice in New York City for twenty-four years, the last fifteen of which have been devoted exclusively to using imagery for treating bodymind problems, including severe chronic illness.